W9-AVL-888

Adult Obesity

Levels of obesity in the UK have tripled over the last 20 years according to a recent report by the National Audit Office. This makes the British among the fattest nations in Europe and, if nothing is done to halt the epidemic, it is feared that levels will soon reach those in the US where one person in every four is obese. Every year tens of thousands of people in the western world are dying prematurely from heart disease, stroke and diabetes – all of them closely linked to obesity.

Obesity is a disease. It is the expression of a classic interaction between nature and nurture. What are the factors responsible for its development? Are we becoming more and more a nation of couch potatoes, or are we just eating too much? Do fat children become fat adults? Can anything be done to halt the obesity epidemic?

This collection of essays, based on a national symposium on obesity, is aimed at the generalist with an interest in managing obesity and its outcomes, whether general practitioner, community nurse, dietician or hospital clinician. Its purpose is to highlight the causes and consequences of obesity and to bring modern understanding to the treatment of a problem that is still heavily stigmatised. The authors offer a wide-ranging perspective of obesity as a global problem and explore its devastating metabolic, social and political impact.

What is increasingly clear is that the seeds of many of these adult diseases are sown in childhood. The prevention of adult obesity has thus become a major challenge for the paediatrician.

Linda Voss is a graduate of the University of St Andrew's, Scotland, and went on to gain a Masters in Education and Psychology. She co-ordinated the long-running Wessex Growth Study for 13 years and has contributed widely to the literature both on childhood growth and psychosocial aspects of short stature. She received her PhD from Southampton in 1998. She is currently Senior Research Fellow at the Peninsula Medical School in Plymouth and Co-ordinator of the EarlyBird Diabetes Study.

Terence Wilkin graduated from St Andrew's Medical School in 1969 and received his MD on thyroid autoimmunity in 1978. Previous posts include: Associate Professor on Endocrinology, University of Montpellier and Wellcome Senior Research Fellow/Reader, University of Southampton. He is a prolific contributor to the literature of thyroid disease, endocrine autoimmunity and osteoporosis. He set up and directed the Wessex Growth Study for a number of years, before moving to Plymouth to set up the EarlyBird Diabetes Study. He is currently Professor of Endocrinology and Metabolism at the Peninsula Medical School, Plymouth, and Honorary Consultant Endocrinologist, Plymouth Hospitals NHS Trust, UK.

Adult Obesity
A paediatric challenge

Edited by
Linda D. Voss and
Terence J. Wilkin

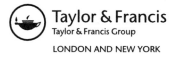

Taylor & Francis
Taylor & Francis Group

LONDON AND NEW YORK

First published 2003
by Taylor & Francis
11 New Fetter Lane, London EC4P 4EE

Simultaneously published in the USA and Canada
by Taylor & Francis
29 West 35th Street, New York, NY 10001

Taylor & Francis is an imprint of the Taylor & Francis Group

Typeset in Baskerville by
HWA Text and Data Management, Tunbridge Wells
Printed and bound in Great Britain by
TJ International Ltd, Padstow, Cornwall

Every effort has been made to ensure that the advice and information in
this book is true and accurate at the time of going to press. However,
neither the publisher nor the authors can accept any legal responsibility
or liability for any errors or omissions that may be made. In the case of
drug administration, any medical procedure or the use of technical
equipment mentioned within this book, you are strongly advised to
consult the manufacturer's guidelines.

British Library Cataloguing in Publication Data
A catalogue record for this book is available from the British Library

Library of Congress Cataloging in Publication Data
Adult obesity : a paediatric challenge / edited by
Terry Wilkin and Linda Voss.
      p. ; cm.
Includes bibliographical references and index.
   1. Obesity–Congresses. 2. Obesity–Etiology–Congresses.
   [DNLM: 1. Obesity–prevention & control–Collected Works.
2. Obesity–prevention & control–Congresses. 3. Health Policy–Collected
Works. 4. Health Policy–Congresses. 5. Obesity–Child–Collected Works.
6. Obesity–Child–Congresses. 7. Obesity–genetics–Collected Works. 8.
Obesity–genetics–Congresses. 9. Primary Health Care–Collected Works.
10. Primary Health Care–Congresses. 11. Self Concept–Collected
Works. 12. Self Concept–Congresses. WD 210 A244 2003] I. Wilkin,
Terry. II. Voss, Linda, 1945–
   RA645.O23 A385 2003
   616.3′98–dc21
                                                                2002151659

ISBN 0–415–30015–0

Contents

ₒ 50767733

Illustrations

Figures

Tables

Contributors

Dr Ian Campbell – Chair of the National Obesity Forum. A Nottingham general practitioner who through the National Obesity Forum has helped to produce the first guidelines for obesity management specifically for primary care. He has developed educational packages and launched a national 'Best Practice' award. He has written several articles and has contributed chapters to two books on obesity management.

Professor Ken Fox – Professor of Exercise and Health Sciences, University of Bristol. Joined the executive of the Association for the Study of Obesity in 1991, and is a former member of the National Audit Office Scientific Advisory Panel on Obesity and the British Nutrition Foundation Task Force on Obesity. He is editor of *The Physical Self: From Motivation to Well-being* and *Physical Activity and Psychological Well-being*.

Professor Philippe Froguel – Professor of Clinical Genetics, Institut Pasteur, Lille. Head of the Department of Human Genetics, Institute of Biology in Lille, France. Professor of Molecular Genetics and Experimental Diabetes at Queen Mary and Westfield College, University of London and Director of the Bart's and London Genomic Centre. He divides his time between Lille and London.

Professor Sir David Hall – President, Royal College of Paediatrics and Child Health. Trained in paediatrics in London, working with the late Dr Hugh Jolly and the child psychiatrist, Dr Emmanuel Lewis. Appointed consultant and senior lecturer in paediatrics to St George's Hospital in 1978, moving in 1993 to become Professor of Community Paediatrics at the University of Sheffield. Was founder and first Chair of the Children's Sub-group of the National Screening Committee and, until 1996, Chair of the Joint Working Parties on Child Health Surveillance. He was elected Vice-President of the Royal College of Paediatrics and Child Health in 1994 and became its President in April 2000.

Dr Andrew Hill – Chair of the Association for the Study of Obesity. Chartered Psychologist and Senior Lecturer in the Division of Psychiatry and Behavioural Sciences at Leeds School of Medicine. He is Associate Fellow of the British Psychological Society, Associate Editor of the *British Journal of Clinical Psychology* and editorial board member of the *International Journal of Obesity*. He has published over ninety academic papers and book chapters.

Professor Philip James – Chair, International Taskforce on Obesity. Following 17 years as Director of the Rowett Research Institute in Aberdeen, he established, and currently chairs, the London headquarters for the International Obesity Taskforce. He chaired the commission on *Nutrition in the 21st Century* for the United Nations and was instrumental in convening a consultation which resulted in a World Health Organization report on the global epidemic of obesity published earlier this year. He is currently lead external scientist for obesity for the World Health Organization.

Ms Suzi Leather – Vice-Chair Food Standards Agency. Appointed to the first Chair of the North and East Devon Health Forum, then to the Chair of Exeter and District Community Health Trust. She is a freelance researcher and writer on consumer aspects of public policy, specializing in health, food and agricultural issues. Ms Leather has worked at regional, national and European level and is a leading national authority on nutrition and poverty.

Professor Terry Wilkin – Professor of Endocrinology and Metabolism, University of Plymouth, and Consultant Endocrinologist. Trained at the Universities of St Andrew's and Montpellier. Wellcome Senior Lecturer and subsequently Reader at Southampton before appointment to the Foundation Chair of Medicine at Plymouth Postgraduate Medical School. Designed and co-supervised, until 1993, the Wessex Growth Study and conducts with Dr Linda Voss the EarlyBird Diabetes Study which aims to better understand the factors in childhood which lead to diabetes.

Preface

Obesity is a disease. It represents a classic interaction between intrinsic susceptibility and environmental risk. The irony is that the genes which survived the ravages of famine during the course of evolution are now deleterious in an industrialized society where food is freely available. The results of this modern epidemic are horrifying. The list of co-morbidities associated with obesity is long – all of them chronic, distressing and costly. Obesity is one of the most important contributors to ill health throughout the world. The World Health Organization, traditionally concerned with under-nutrition, now recognizes that obesity contributes more to malnutrition, worldwide, than under-nutrition. Yet many still fail to recognize obesity as a disease, regarding the patient as culpable and the issue as social rather than medical.

This collection of essays is based on the presentations made to a national symposium on obesity, held under the auspices of the new Peninsula Medical School at Plymouth in May 2001. It draws together some of the greatest expertise in the country and covers a considerable amount of ground. Like the symposium on which it is based, the book is not intended for the expert. Rather, it is aimed at the clinician, nurse, dietitian or administrator who has an interest in understanding more about the problem of obesity, the mechanisms responsible and the impact it has on individuals and on society. The title of the collection, *Adult Obesity, a Paediatric Challenge*, encapsulates its thrust. Obesity and its metabolic impact start in childhood. Those who suffer as adults from the complications of obesity are more likely to have been obese as children. The incidence of obesity in today's children is nearly three times what it was just a generation ago and, even at the age of 5 years, its impact is measurable on the markers of metabolic and cardiovascular disease which we know spell danger for adults.

The book opens with a global perspective from Professor Philip James, Chairman of the International Obesity Taskforce. Global data make clear the extraordinary scale of the current obesity epidemic. We tend to think of

North America as the worst affected, but this is far from being the case. Professor Ken Fox then highlights the appallingly low levels of physical activity in our modern lifestyle and suggests that physical activity contributes more to the obesity epidemic than change in calorie consumption.

Professor Philippe Froguel, a formidable geneticist working both sides of the English Channel, summarizes the rapid development of our understanding of how genes control appetite, fat distribution and insulin resistance. Professor Terry Wilkin (Plymouth) discusses the environmental and lifestyle factors which may lead to insulin resistance – one of the main mechanisms whereby obesity impacts on metabolic health. He uses the EarlyBird Diabetes Study of healthy young school entrants to illustrate how early in life the process of insulin resistance begins, and concludes with a challenge to the paediatricians, inviting a response from the President of the Royal College of Paediatrics and Child Health.

There are many agencies in government concerned with the rising epidemic of obesity, and Suzi Leather, Vice-Chair of the Food Standards Agency, summarizes the remit of her own Agency and the position it takes over strategies to close the ever widening 'nutrition gap' in our society. The next two chapters continue the theme of threats and opportunities in the management of obesity. Dr Andrew Hill, Chair of the Association for the Study of Obesity, explores the impact of obesity on self-esteem and the stigma commonly attached to it. He concludes with a provoking discussion of responsibility and blame. On a more optimistic note, Dr Ian Campbell, Chair of the National Obesity Forum, shows what can be achieved in general practice, where most cases will first present, given the commitment and enthusiasm of the primary care team.

Professor Sir David Hall, President of the Royal College of Paediatrics and Child Health, concludes with a practical as well as a political view of obesity. He acknowledges obesity to be a major public health issue and, in spite of the enormous difficulties involved in tackling the problem, accepts that it is one that paediatricians can no longer afford to ignore.

As a clinical, rather than cosmetic problem, obesity is only now beginning to emerge in the UK, and what is seen today is only the first ripple of an impending tidal wave. *The Plymouth Symposium on Obesity and Insulin Resistance* has become an annual event. It seems likely that interest in this area of medicine will continue to dominate the health agenda for the foreseeable future.

Linda Voss
Terry Wilkin

Acknowledgements

We are indebted to Laurie Barron, Corrina Mossop and Jacqueline Pearson for their help in the preparation of these manuscripts.

Part I
The issue

1 Obesity: a global problem

Philip James

Introduction

The first ever report on obesity by the World Health Organization (WHO) was published in December 2000 (World Health Organization, 2000). It was based on an expert technical consultation, which convened in 1997, after a draft report had been produced by the International Obesity TaskForce (IOTF) with its eleven subcommittees of experts from across the world. Originally, WHO had not considered obesity important because its role, in particular, was to help the developing world, and it was assumed that obesity only affected affluent societies. The prevailing prejudice that individuals were to blame for over-indulging themselves or being slothful clearly influenced WHO officials' rejection of the problem. This approach was in no way unusual. Obesity has long been considered of little importance by doctors, who usually find their obese patients difficult to manage and concerned about what seems to be a cosmetic problem. In practice, it has now become clear that we are in the middle of a global epidemic of an important disease affecting both children and adults. The challenge now is to produce coherent data to highlight the problem and seek solutions for its prevention and management.

In the mid 1990s, WHO undertook an evaluation of underweight and overweight in both children and adults (World Health Organization, 1995). At that stage the problem of chronic energy deficiency in adults was being recognized for the first time (James *et al.*, 1988), but when representative data were obtained from a number of countries it soon became evident that underweight or 'chronic energy deficiency' of adults was comparatively unusual and that many developing countries had a far greater problem of excess weight (Figure 1.1). For this analysis the standard measure of body mass index (BMI, kg/m^2) was used and, in order to accommodate the problem of underweight in adults, it was recognized that the lower limit of the normal range of BMI should be extended to 18.5 (Table 1.1).

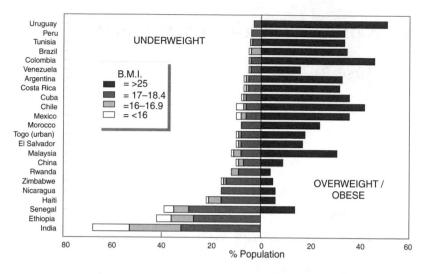

Figure 1.1 BMI distribution of adult population from surveys worldwide. Reproduced with permission from WHO (2000).

Table 1.1 WHO classification of obesity (BMI = weight (kg)/height (m)²)

WHO classification	BMI	Risk of co-morbidity
Underweight	Below 18.5	Low
Healthy weight	18.5–24.9	Average
Overweight (grade1 obesity)	25.0–29.9	Mild increase
Obese (grade 2 obesity)	30.0–39.0	Moderate/severe
Morbid/severe obesity (grade 3)	40.0 and above	Very severe

WHO. *Obesity: Preventing and Managing the Global Epidemic.* Geneva: WHO, 1997[3].

The problem with only worrying about individuals categorized as overweight if their BMI is over 25.0, and coping medically with patients as 'obese' once they have a BMI of 30.0 or more, neglects the fact that there is a distribution of BMIs within the population and that, as the epidemic grows, the whole population's distribution of BMIs is shifting upwards. Thus there is an extraordinary increase in obesity rates with seemingly modest increases in the average BMI of a population (Rose, 1991). In the early 1980s, China had a beautiful gaussian distribution of BMIs with an average of about 21, and only a small proportion of underweight and overweight adults. Compare this with the United States, where the average BMI of the population is over 25 and obesity rates are currently 30 per cent or more. These countries display the two extremes of a spectrum, but it is now clear that a dramatic shift to the right is occurring with escalating obesity rates throughout the world.

The disease burden of obesity

The hazards of a weight increase have been underestimated because, traditionally, epidemiologists have simply regarded weight gain as one of the risk factors affecting blood pressure, the propensity to diabetes and dyslipidaemia. Thus the risks of cardiovascular disease were ascribed to hypertension and dyslipidaemia, rather than to an underlying driver, that is, unhealthy weight gain. What is now evident is that, even within the so-called normal range of BMI, there is a markedly increased risk of type 2 diabetes as BMI rises. The risk is minimal when BMIs are held at about 20 and with no weight increase in adult life. By the time adults have reached a BMI of 25, both men and women have a five- to six-fold increased risk of diabetes and this risk escalates further at higher levels of BMI (Willett *et al.*, 1999). The risk of hypertension also rises rapidly but one of the most intriguing features is the progressive reduction in blood high-density lipoprotein (HDL) cholesterol levels once the BMI starts rising above about 20. A low HDL cholesterol is one of the most powerful predictors of the risk of coronary heart disease and Shaper and colleagues, conducting the British Regional Heart Survey (Shaper *et al.*, 1997), found marked falls in HDL with substantial increases in total cholesterol, serum triglycerides and blood pressure in adult men even before they were outside the normal BMI range. By the time British middle-aged men reach BMIs of 30, a third of them have hypertension.

New approaches to assessing the burden of disease linked to obesity are now being published. A recent Australian study (Mathers *et al.*, 1999) assessed the total burden of disease in terms of the number of years of life lost and the number of years lived in a disabled state (disability adjusted life years or DALYs), and assessed the likely contributors to the major diseases affecting Victoria state in Australia. Figure 1.2 reveals that diet and physical inactivity account for a greater burden than that imposed by tobacco and, even in these analyses, the burden from obesity was arbitrarily halved to take account of the potential impact of physical inactivity in precipitating overweight and obesity. The same study also showed that the burden of disease expressed in DALYs increased with age and became substantial in middle-aged women.

Martorell *et al.* (2000) recently assessed the overall prevalence of overweight and obesity in women from different parts of the world, and the extent of the global epidemic is very clear. Although North American women

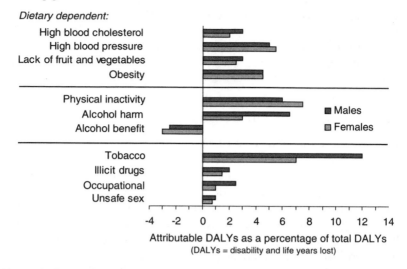

Figure 1.2 Proportion of total burden of disease attributable to selected risk factors, by sex, Australia 1996 (Source: Mathers *et al.*, 1999).

have major problems of obesity, to everyone's surprise, the overall figures are matched by those from the ex-command economies, that is, Eastern Europe and the former Soviet Union, and *exceeded* by the rates of overweight and obesity in women living in the Middle East. The IOTF has been conducting similar analyses on men as well as women, and estimates that there are about 315 million obese adults in the world and about three-quarters of a billion who are overweight. This therefore represents an extraordinary disease burden.

Asian sensitivities to obesity-related morbidity

Although Asians are classified, using standard WHO criteria, as not having an appreciable problem of obesity, a group of experts led by Professors Zimmet and Inoue from Australia and Japan, met in Hong Kong under the auspices of WHO, the International Association for the Study of Obesity (IASO) and the IOTF. On the basis of their assessments of preliminary data from Hong Kong and Japan, they suggested that adult Asians could no longer be classified in BMI terms in the same way as the rest of the world (WHO/IASO/IOTF, 2000). They proposed that in people of Asian origin the upper limit of a normal BMI should be 23, and that a BMI of 25 should trigger the diagnosis of obesity. This new development is obviously contentious because, hitherto, when dealing with children's growth, the WHO has studiously avoided considering local growth standards, particularly when it became evident that Third World children brought up in a hygienic, well-fed and nurturing environment grew at rates equivalent to WHO standards.

The question, therefore, is whether people of Asian origin are genetically different, or whether they simply display an unusual sensitivity to diabetes and hypertension because of some prevailing nutritional or other environmental problem. It is clear, however, that there are differences between ethnic groups in their susceptibility to diabetes. This could reflect not only the impact of environmental factors such as diet on insulin resistance, but also the effects of dietary and other factors which alter the pancreatic capacity to secrete insulin. Type 2 diabetes emerges when the pancreatic capacity is unable to meet the long-standing demands made when overweight and obese adults develop insulin resistance and require a far greater endogenous output of insulin from the pancreas as it ages. Comparable data on the propensity to diabetes in adults with measured glucose intolerance have now shown that Scandinavian Caucasians have a rate of developing type 2 diabetes of about 5–6 per cent per year. In China, however, the comparable value, despite lower BMIs, is a 15 per cent conversion rate per year (Pen *et al.*, 1997) These differences are mirrored by clear evidence that Mexican Americans and Hispanics have much greater prevalences of diabetes at the same body weights as white Americans living in the United States (Edelstein *et al.*, 1997).

Early influences on adult disease

It has been well recognized that adults are much more liable to develop diabetes if they were already obese in childhood and entered adult life in an obese state. Further weight gain in adult life, which is then likely, amplifies the risk and it becomes 80- to 100-fold greater than that observed in adults who mature with a BMI of 20 and gain no further weight. This is a clear demonstration of the importance of early adiposity in precipitating the onset of type 2 diabetes (Colditz, 1995). Earlier risk factors are also evident: babies born to diabetic mothers tend not only to be larger than normal, but also to have a much greater propensity to developing type 2 diabetes, even in adolescence.

More intriguing, however, is the increasing evidence that fetal exposure to poor maternal nutrition may alter the pancreatic capacity of the child to cope subsequently. Barker (1994) has developed an hypothesis, based on very coherent experimental animal data, showing that animals born to mothers whose diet has been restricted in protein have pancreatic changes which reduce their capacity to generate insulin, and hepatic structural alter-ations which change gluconeogenesis and cholesterol metabolism. In primates as well as rodents it has been clearly demonstrated that the maternal diet and/or immediate post-natal diet can permanently alter the sensitivity of the offspring in terms of cholesterol metabolism and long-term body size. Barker proposed that analogous conditions occurred in man, and that babies born small were particularly likely to display higher blood pressure, a propensity to diabetes and coronary heart disease some 50 to 60 years later. This hypothesis was considered controversial because it might wrongly be implied that the children were doomed to chronic adult disease when in fact the experimental data suggest that the fetal changes mainly affect the propensity to respond to dietary and other changes in late life. Nevertheless, in his original studies of Hertfordshire men, Barker showed a progressive increase in the risk of abdominal obesity and the metabolic syndrome of diabetes, high blood pressure and abnormal lipids, the lower the weight of the men at birth.

There is also increasing evidence of an association between small babies and stunted growth in early childhood (James *et al.*, 2000) and stunting has now been clearly linked to a greater likelihood of developing abdominal obesity and the metabolic syndrome in later life (Schroeder *et al.*, 1999). A plausible hypothesis is that poor fetal nutrition limits the placenta's capacity to metabolize circulating maternal cortisol. This then passes to the fetus, thereby amplifying fetal cortisol levels and resetting the fetal hypothalamic pituitary adrenal axis. Thus there may be subtle hypercorticolism induced by fetal experiences which, as seen in clinical Cushing's disease, alters the distribution of fat, channelling it to the abdomen. Here, it is considered to be particularly hazardous perhaps, in part, because a large release of fatty acids then enters the portal circulation which normally does not carry an excess to the liver.

Data from India now reveal that although about a third of babies are born small with low birth weight (<2.5 kg), they have an additional handicap in that they already have, probably because of poor maternal diets, less lean tissue and more body fat than normal. If they subsequently grow well, these small babies, by the age of 8 years, already display higher blood pressures and insulin resistance than normal children (Yajnik, 2000). Indians, whether in India or the UK, have a greater propensity to abdominal obesity, and 12 per cent of Indian adults in the Indian slums are diabetic, with a further 18 per cent glucose intolerant. This extraordinary epidemic of diabetes is occurring when adults have BMIs of only 23 or 24.

Among a total of some 400 million Indian city dwellers there is already a massive, largely unrecognized, public health problem. Glucose-intolerant and diabetic young women are, in turn, likely to produce babies with a greater propensity to diabetes. We seem to be witnessing a major intergenerational shift in programming of extraordinary consequence. If one considers the analogous data from the Caribbean, South Africa and

Latin America, with preliminary suggestions that the more disadvantaged Chinese are also affected, then we appear to have an extraordinary synergy between fetal and childhood malnutrition and adult chronic disease. The implication is that well over half the world is currently born with a greater propensity to early cardiovascular disease and marked sensitivities to the co-morbidities associated with only quite modest weight gains.

Childhood poverty and obesity: a cause for concern

It must be recognized that the original work on the association between events in pregnancy and adult health care came from Scandinavia and the UK. More recent reports from Finland again show that the combination of a low birth weight and poor early growth in the babe during the first year of life, followed by more rapid weight gain in childhood, is particularly deleterious. If the mother's BMI at term is particularly high, the offspring have an additional handicap. This raises major questions about the need to consider intervention studies. It is now estimated that between 60 and 90 per cent of all the world's diabetes is precipitated by excess weight gain. Excess weight gain is also now being highlighted as a major contributor to the massive public health problem of hypertension evident in both the developed world and Asia.

In Britain we have underestimated the importance of obesity and its underlying causes. It is now evident (see Figure 1.3) that children are displaying rapid increases in the prevalence of both overweight and obesity, this epidemic having accelerated from the mid-1980s (Bundred *et al.*, 2001). New unpublished analyses from across the world indicate a similar epidemic occurring in the developing world as well. This is leading to huge changes in policy. In Chile, for example, there have been multi-billion dollar payments for decades in order to provide food supplements for poor children with stunted growth. These supplements payments are now in the process of being withdrawn because it has been discovered that these children show a remarkable propensity to obesity and are not being helped by the additional provision of fats and sugars! Chile is now confronted with a rising tide of disease which is particularly apparent in the poorer communities and linked to overweight and obesity. We are therefore seeing a rapid transition, right across the world, from the original societal view that obesity was an index of affluence and wellbeing to a clear recognition that obesity is associated with poverty and the disadvantaged sectors of society (Pena and Bacallao, 2000).

Since childhood obesity is clearly a forerunner of adult problems, we have now entered an extraordinary new era. Never before in the history of mankind have we seen, within a single generation, a transformation in the

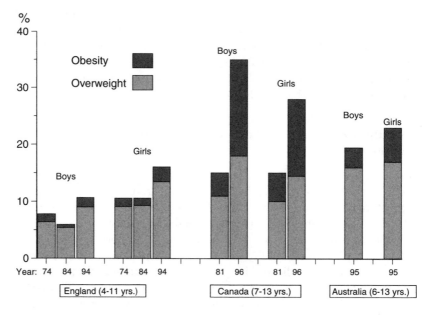

Figure 1.3 The increasing prevalence of overweight and obesity in children. The UK and Australian analyses are based on the use of the IOTF cut-off points set out by Cole *et al.* (2000) whereas the Canadian data make use of the 85th and 95th percentile values of the US standardized curves. UK data: Chinn and Rona, 2001; Canadian data: Tremblay and Willms, 2000; Australian data: Booth *et al.*, 2001.

health priorities of children. From an obsession with children as the vulnerable group, liable to malnutrition, we are now having to rethink our whole approach to societal circumstances, the upbringing of children and how best to prevent overweight and obesity with its alarming long-term consequences.

References

Barker, D.J.P. (1994) *Mothers, Babies and Disease in Later Life*. London: BMJ Publishing Group.

Booth, M.L., Wake, M., Armstrong, T., Chey, T., Hesketh, K. and Mathur, S. (2001) The epidemiology of overweight and obesity among Australian children and adolescents, 1995–97. *Aust N Z J Public Health*, 25(2): 162–9.

Bundred, P., Kitchiner, D. and Buchan, I. (2001) Prevalence of overweight and obese children between 1989 and 1998: population based series of cross sectional studies, *Brit Med J*, 322: 326–8.

Chinn, S. and Rona, R.J. (2001) Prevalence and trends in overweight and obesity in three cross sectional studies of British children, 1974–94. *Br Med J*, 322: 24–6.

Colditz, G.A., Willett, W.C., Rotnitzky, A. and Manson, J.E. (1995) Weight gain as a risk factor for clinical diabetes mellitus in women, *Ann Intern Med*, 122(7): 481–6.

Cole, T.J., Bellizzi, M.C., Flegal, K.M. and Dietz, W.H. (2000) Establishing a standard definition for child overweight and obesity worldwide international survey. *Br Med J*, 320: 1240–3.

Edelstein, S.L., Knowler, W.C., Bain, R.P., Andres, R., Barrett-Connor, E.L., Dowse, G.K., Haffner, S.M., Pettitt, D., Sorkin, I.D., Muller, D.C., Collins, V.R. and Haimnan, R.E. (1997) Predictors of progression from impaired glucose tolerance to NIDDM: an analysis of six prospective studies, *Diabetes*, 46(4): 701–10.

James, W.P.T., Ferro-Luzzi, A. and Waterlow, J.C.(1988) Definition of chronic energy deficiency in adults. Report of a Working Party of the International Dietary Energy Consultative Group. *Eur J of Chin Nutr*, 42(12): 969–81.

James, W.P.T., Norum, K., Smitasiri, S., Swaminathan, M.S., Tagwiiye, I., Uauy, R. and Ul-Haq, M. (2000) *Ending Malnutrition by 2020: An Agenda for Change in the Millennium.* Final Report to the ACC/SCN by the Commission on the Nutrition Challenges of the 21st Century. Supplement to the Food and Nutrition Bulletin, 2000. UNU International Nutrition Foundation, USA.

Martorell, R., Kettel Klian, L., Hughes, M.L. and Grununer-Strawn, L.M. (2000) Obesity in women from developing countries. *European Journal of Clinical Nutrition*, 54: 247–52.

Mathers, C., Vos, T. and Stevenson, C. (1999) The burden of disease and injury in Australia, AIHW cat. no PHE 17, Canberra: AIHW.

Pan, X.-R., Li, G.-W., Hu, Y.-H *et al.*(1997) Effects of diet and exercise in preventing NIDDM in people with impaired glucose tolerance. The Da Qing IGT and Diabetes Study. *Diabetes Care*, 20: 537–44.

Pena, M. and Bacallao, I. (eds) (2000) Obesity and poverty. *Pan American Health Organization Scientific Publication*, 576: 41–9.

Rose, G. (1991) Population distributions of risk and disease, *Nutr Metab Cardiovasc Dis*, 1: 37–40.

Schroeder, D.G., Martorell, R. and Flores, R.(1999) Infant and child growth and fatness and fat distribution in Guatemalan adults. *Am J Epidemiol*, 149(2): 177–85.

Shaper, A.G., Wannamethee, S.G. and Walker, M. (1997) Body weight: implications for the prevention of coronary heart disease, stroke, and diabetes mellitus in a cohort study of middle aged men, *Br Med J*, 314: 1311–17.

Tremblay, M.S. and Willms, J.D. (2000) Secular trends in the body mass index of Canadian children. *Can Med Assoc J*, 163:1429–33.

WHO/IASO/IOTF (2000) *The Asia-Pacific Perspective: Redefining Obesity and its Treatment.* Full document available from: http://www.idi.org.au/obesity-report.htm.

Willett, W., Dietz, W. and Colditz, G.A.(1999) Guidelines for healthy weight. *N Engl J Med*, 341: 427–34.

12   *Philip James*

World Health Organization (1995) *Physical Status: The Use and Interpretation of Anthropometry.* WHO Technical Report, series no. 854. Geneva: World Health Organization.

World Health Organization (2000) *Obesity: Preventing and Managing the Global Epidemic.* WHO Technical Report, series no. 894. Geneva: World Health Organization.

Yajnik, C. (2000) Interactions of perturbations in intrauterine growth and growth during childhood on the risk of adult-onset disease. *Proc Nut Soc,* 59: 1–9.

2 Underactivity or overnutrition?

Ken Fox

Obesity is a problem of the new millennium: I doubt that we have seen an epidemic like this since the plague. The question we have to ask is, why is it happening? While nutrition and exercise are clearly both important, I should declare a bias because I am an exercise, not a nutritional specialist. I will therefore be focusing mainly on the subject of physical activity, but I think I can provide good reason for doing so.

Homo erectus is relatively new on the scene in terms of geological time – it took us several million years to evolve to modern man – but in just the last 20 years or so we in the western world have seen a dramatic change in our physical dimensions. Something serious has happened to our body shape that cannot be explained by genetic changes. Although some people clearly have a genetic predisposition to acquire weight, it takes a long period to shift the gene pool itself. The change seen over the last 20 years must be related to energy balance. We are either eating too much for our level of activity or we are not sufficiently active for the amount we eat. We have to look at both sides of the equation together, as they clearly interact.

Eating is easy

Our present situation could be described as a poor evolutionary adaptation to a rapidly shifting culture – we are ill-equipped to deal with the environment that we have created for ourselves. There are strong signals to eat and very weak signals to stop. Most of us get hungry very quickly and there is certainly increased availability of food, 24 hours a day. We are adapted to eat as much as we can and, indeed, we often overeat, especially when we are celebrating and have an excuse to do so. Eating is very rewarding – we build a lot of our social activities into eating and drinking and it is pleasurable. There is also no viable alternative to eating – we need to eat to survive.

Eating well is also regarded as high status – we like to go to nice restaurants and spend money on good food. Physiologically, psychologically and sociologically, we are encouraged to eat.

Exercise is hard

The opposite is true for activity. Here, the signal is weak and it takes an effort to get up and move. There is evidence of this in the animal kingdom, where lions will only stir themselves when hungry and then just use a short burst of energy to seek and catch food. There are certainly strong signals to stop being energetic. Physical activity can hurt if you have not done it for a while – it makes you sweaty, and it makes your heart race. These sensations can become mentally exhilarating with experience, but those unaccustomed to exercise are easily put off. Inactivity, on the other hand, can be rewarding. After a hard day's work at the computer, we come home and treat ourselves by putting our feet up and opening a can of beer. Inactivity is a viable alternative and, in the short term, we can get away with it. It is the long-term consequences that are so negative to health. Inactivity is also high status. We like having two cars in the drive and we like to surround ourselves by energy saving devices. These are signals that we are wealthy and doing very well in society. This modern lifestyle of ample food and easy living is not going to disappear overnight, and we have to find ways of dealing with the problem now. The question is, to what extent does overeating or lack of physical activity explain the rapid increase in obesity?

Are we eating more or exercising less?

According to the Health Surveys of England, while obesity has been steadily rising over the last few decades, there does not appear to have been a corresponding change in energy intake or fat intake (Figure 2.1) (Prentice and Jebb, 1995). In contrast, the rise in number of cars per household and TV hours watched per week would suggest increasing inactivity is to blame. These data, however, rely on self-report to estimate food consumption. It is difficult to estimate, precisely, how much people actually consume. There is a tendency, especially among diet-conscious younger people, to under-report. A US survey, however, isolated data from an elderly population, where under-reporting would have been less likely, and showed no change in self-reported energy intake in spite of a significant rise in levels of obesity. Consumption of fat appears, if anything, to be falling, although the same caveat as above must apply to estimates of fat intake based on self-report. Further data do, however, indicate that consumption of low-calorie products is rising, which suggests that people are becoming more health-conscious. Such food intake data cannot explain the current rise in obesity.

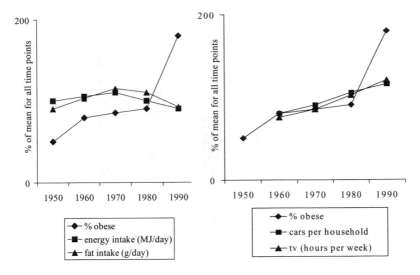

Figure 2.1 Secular trends in diet and acitivity in relation to obesity in Britain (Source: Prentice and Jebb, 1995).

Energy expenditure and the modern lifestyle

We come back to inactivity. Modern technology is changing our world. Jobs are largely sedentary, buildings are equipped with lifts and escalators, we own more cars, demand cheaper petrol, and our homes are full of labour-saving devices. We are surrounded by screen technology and wall-to-wall entertainment. Most children have a television in their bedroom. All these compete with energy expenditure. Our present environment is not conducive to an active lifestyle, and this major cultural shift has imposed further restrictions on society. Parents, women and older people are increasingly worried about the real or perceived dangers outside the home. It has been estimated that the difference in energy expenditure today, compared to an earlier generation, might be some 300 to 500 calories per day (World Health Organization, 1995). Given this decrease in energy expenditure, it would only take a susceptible person some seven to ten days to put on 1 lb of fat.

Small changes in energy expenditure can thus make a big difference. Contrary to popular perception, 'fitness fanatics' are few and far between, belonging largely to the middle or professional classes. In a recent survey, a substantial proportion of the population confessed to having indulged in no vigorous, or even moderate, physical activity in the previous month (Figure 2.2), (Health Education Authority/Sports Council, 1992). Moreover, the percentage rose with increasing age, mirroring the inexorable age-related rise in obesity.

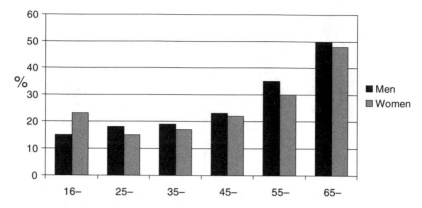

Figure 2.2 Population percentage reporting no moderate or vigorous activity in previous month (Source: HEA/Sports Council, 1992).

Childhood obesity

Turning our attention to children, we face a similar challenge. Our levels of childhood obesity are rising and so too are the number of paediatric referrals (Flegal, 1999; Reilly and Dorosty, 1999). The health implications are already clear – 60 per cent of overweight children have at least one risk factor for coronary heart disease. So called 'adult-onset diabetes' is increasingly appearing in adolescents and early-onset obesity also increases the chances of obesity tracking into adulthood (Barlow and Dietz, 1998). The earlier you are a fat child, and the longer you are a fat child, the greater your risk of becoming a fat adult. When this first generation of fatter children appears in the health statistics in 20 years' time, the present figures will be seen as relatively mild. Having said that, only 30 per cent of obese adults today were obese as children. Many people become fat later in life, so prevention of childhood obesity is only part of the solution.

Falling activity levels in childhood

The number of children who walk to school is diminishing and the number driven by car increasing (Department of Environment, Transport, and the Regions, 1997). Fewer than 10 per cent of children cycle to school in the UK. Cycling has never been popular and is not encouraged by the shortage of bicycle sheds at school. In Holland the figure is close to 70 per cent and this is reflected in a lower prevalence of obesity. Apart from the fact that they have no hills, the Dutch have the advantage of bicycle lanes beside every road, making cycling both easier and safer. Physical education as provided in school does little to help. Our provision is among the worst in Europe and our children spend less than one per cent of their waking time in physical education. Even if we were to increase the time allocated to it, it would do little to solve the energy expenditure problem that children face, given the hours they spend in front of their televisions, computers and play stations. Children actually do very little activity out of school. Forty per cent of younger boys say they play football (Gregory, 2000). Over the age of 14, a similar percentage say they just walk. Girls report even less activity – the older ones report walking to be their main activity, followed by 'cleaning'!

Is overprotection to blame?

Figures showing the percentage of children who actually achieve health education authority recommendations for physical activity make appalling reading. Around 60 per cent of 7- to14-year-old boys manage to undertake about an hour's moderate activity per day (Gregory, 2000). This drops to a little over 40 per cent by 15–18 years. Girls fare even less well. Only around 40 per cent achieve the target at 7–14 years of age, this figure falling to 30 per cent by the time they are in their teens. One explanation for these figures is likely to be the change, in recent years, in parental licence for children to go out alone, whether to play, to go to the shops or to ride a bike. One report suggests that the 10-year-old of today is only allowed the freedom previously granted to a 7-year-old (Hillman, 1993). There is also a gender difference, relating no doubt to parental anxiety, which may, in part, explain the lower levels of physical activity generally found in girls. There certainly seems to be a tendency for children today to be closeted and protected for their own safety. Are we creating a generation of 'battery' instead of 'free-range' kids?

Measuring physical activity

Self-report is unreliable, both for dietary intake and for patterns of physical activity. Instead, we have made use of little gadgets called CSA accelerometers that attach to the belt and record all movement. The data can subsequently be downloaded to display minute-by-minute patterns of physical activity during the day. These devices show that girls, in comparison with boys, have lower levels of physical activity at school (unpublished data, Department of Health Sciences, Bristol University). They run around less at breaktime. Boys appear to be less active out of school and at weekends. We have just completed a study comparing a school week to a half-term week. It used to be the case that, during the holidays, children would play outside from dawn to dusk. Nowadays, it seems, children are even less active in holiday time than they are in the school week (unpublished data, Department of Health Sciences, Bristol University). The school day is therefore of critical importance in ensuring that some physical activity takes place. Girls are not less active in the holidays, largely because they are very inactive all the time! We also compared obese with normal-weight boys; the obese boys tended to be less active at each point of the school day and by the end of the day, were really slowing down (unpublished data, Department of Health Sciences, Bristol University). Their lower levels of activity were even clearer at the weekend. We cannot be sure that inactivity led to the obesity in the first instance, but it does appear that obese boys are likely to be perpetuating their condition through inactivity. They are late risers, for example, especially on a Sunday morning. Clearly, this is one area where there is scope for intervention. The girls' data did not show a significant difference between obese and non-obese children, probably because the non- obese girls were so low in activity themselves. Curiously, obese girls seemed to become more active on weekend afternoons – perhaps they are making a conscious effort to exercise.

The two obvious ways of tackling obesity are to eat less and to exercise more. There are risks associated with the former, especially in teenage girls, because some, especially those who suffer from a fear of fatness, do not eat enough to maintain a healthy nutrient status (Gregory, 2000). This is a group at high risk of malnutrition, and it might be helpful if we were to focus less on nutrition and more on the effectiveness of physical activity.

Does physical activity improve health in the overweight and the obese?

There is good evidence that activity is good for your health, no matter your size. Physical activity offers the same protection to the overweight and obese as it does those of normal weight (Figure 2.3) (Lee *et al.*, 1999). Inactivity should really be regarded as a risk factor for coronary heart disease in the same way as smoking, hypertension and high cholesterol. Highly active people, even those with several well-recognized risk factors, have similar levels of mortality to those with no obvious risk factors but who do no exercise (US Department of Health and Human Services (PHS), 1996). They may be relatively rare, but fat people who exercise can reduce their risk to a level similar to those who are slightly overweight and even of normal weight. It is not possible to assess a person's risk simply by looking at them – it is of crucial importance to know how active they are. On an encouraging note, the data clearly show that it is never too late to adopt an active lifestyle. Middle-aged people who remain fit over a 5-year period have a 70 per cent reduction in mortality compared to those who remain unfit over the same period, but even those who move from the unfit to the fit category can halve their risk (Blair *et al.*, 1995).

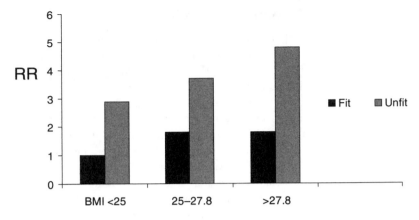

Figure 2.3 Relative risk of CVD mortality by BMI group (Source: Lee *et al.*, 1999).

Does physical activity assist weight loss?

Exercise alone will only produce, on average, a weight loss of around 0.5 kg a month and is less effective than dietary restriction alone (Fox and Page, 2001). The two together will give the best results. The real value of exercise, however, lies in the fact that muscle tissue is preserved and the proportion of weight lost as fat increases. The benefits of exercise are, therefore, much longer term.

Does physical activity help maintain weight loss?

Data comparing diet and exercise programmes show that those who continue to exercise maintain their weight loss (Pavlou *et al.*, 1989). It is very rare for long-term weight loss to be sustained without some physical activity in the process.

Can physical activity prevent weight gain?

There is a tendency for people to put on weight as they age and there are good cross-sectional data showing that those who are physically active, whether through walking, cycling, playing golf or running, can slow this process down (Di Pietro, 1999). Prospective data confirm the benefits of activity in preventing weight gain (Di Pietro *et al.*, 1998; Coakley *et al.*, 1998). The risk, for example, of putting on a significant amount of weight over a period of 10 years is hugely increased in women who remain inactive (Williamson *et al.*, 1993).

Does inactivity help maintain weight gain?

It is increasingly clear that inactivity – the time spent sitting down watching TV or at the computer – is as important as physical activity, and a clear association can be seen between BMI and the hours spend in sedentary pursuits (Jebb and Moore, 1999).

In summary, whatever the relative importance ascribed to underactivity and overnutrition, there is a paediatric problem that needs to be addressed. The focus to date has been largely on overnutrition, and it is to be hoped that future research will attempt to redress the balance a little. Some fortunate children seem to be able to get away with eating large amounts without gaining weight. Others clearly have a genetic susceptibility to putting on weight. Importantly, those who have a high energy intake and are inactive are those most at risk of obesity. It is important that we are aware of the interaction between all these factors in each and every child.

References

Barlow, S.E. and Dietz, W.H. (1998) Obesity evaluation and treatment: expert committee recommendations. *Pediatrics*, 102: E29.

Blair, S.N., Kohl, H.W., Barlow, C.E. *et al.* (1995) Changes in physical fitness and all-cause mortality: a prospective study of healthy and unhealthy men. *JAMA*, 273: 1093–8.

Coakley, E.H., Rimm, E.B., Colditz, G., Kawachi, I. and Willett, W. (1998) Predictors of weight change in men: results from The Health Professionals Follow-Up Study. *Int J Obes*, 22: 89–96.

Department of Environment, Transport, and the Regions (1997) *Walking in Great Britain*. London: The Stationery Office.

DiPietro, L. (1999) Physical activity in the prevention of obesity: current evidence and research issues. *Med Sci Sport Exerc*, 31: S542–6.

Di Pietro, L., Kohl, H.W., Barlow, C.E. and Blair, S.N. (1998) Improvements in cardiorespiratory fitness attenuate age-related weight gain in healthy men and women: the Aerobics Centre Longitudinal Study. *Int J Obes*, 22: 55–62.

Flegal, K.M. (1999) The obesity epidemic in children and adults: current evidence and research issues. *Med Sci Sports Exerc*, 31: S509–14.

Fox, K.R. and Page, A. (2001) The physical activity approach to the treatment of overweight and obesity. In P. Kopelman (ed.) *The Management of Obesity and Related Disorders*. London: Dunitz.

Gregory, J. (2000) *The National Dietary and Nutrition Survey for 4–18 Year Olds*. London: The Stationery Office.

Health Education Authority and Sports Council (1992) *Allied Dunbar National Fitness Survey: Main Findings*. London: Author.

Hillman, M. (1993) One false move. In M. Hillman (ed.) *Children, Transport and Quality of Life*, pp. 7–18. London: Policy Studies Institute.

Jebb, S.A. and Moore, M.S. (1999) Contribution of a sedentary lifestyle and inactivity to the etiology of overweight and obesity: current evidence and research issues. *Med Sci Sport Exerc*, 31: S534–41.

Lee, C.D., Blair, S.N., and Jackson, A.S. (1999) Cardiorespiratory fitness, body composition, and all-cause mortality in men. *Am J Clin Nutr*, 69: 373–80.

Pavlou, K.N., Krey, S. and Steffee, W.P. (1989) Exercise as an adjunct to weight loss and maintenance in moderately obese subjects. *Am J Clin Nutr*, 49: 1115–23.

Prentice, A.M. and Jebb, S. (1995) Obesity in Britain: gluttony or sloth. *Br Med J*, 311: 437–9.

Reilly, J.J. and Dorosty, A.H. (1999) Epidemic of obesity in UK children. *Lancet*, 354: 1874–5.

US Department of Health and Human Services (PHS) (1996) *Physical Activity and Health*. A report of the Surgeon General (Executive Summary), Superintendent of Documents, Pittsburgh, PA.

Williamson, D.F., Madans, J., Anda, R.F., Kleinman, J.C., Kahn, H.S. and Byers, T. (1993) Recreational physical activity and ten-year weight change in a US national cohort. *Int J Obes*, 17: 279–86.

World Health Organization (1995) Exercise for health. WHO/FIMS Committee on Physical Activity for Health. *Bull World Health Organization*, 73: 135–6.

Part II

Nature and nurture

3   Do our genes make us fat?

Philippe Froguel

Introduction

Obesity is a common disorder that has become more prevalent in all countries over the past few years (World Health Organization, 1997). About 10 per cent of the French population, 17–20 per cent of the English and Welsh and over 25 per cent of North Americans are obese (Maillard *et al.*, 2000; Prescott-Clarke and Primatesta, 1998; World Health Organization, 1997). In Europe, although obesity is less prevalent in adults than in the US, the prevalence of overweight is increasing among children and teenagers. In France, the most recent data show that 16 per cent of children and teenagers are overweight and the number of obese children has increased five-fold in the last 10 years (Maillard *et al.*, 2000). Obesity is a risk factor for early death and a wide range of metabolic and cardiovascular complications (Lean *et al.*, 1998).

Although rapid globalization of the Westernised way of life is responsible for the outstanding rise in the prevalence of obesity (about 1 billion people are now overweight or frankly obese), obesity is a typical, common, multifactorial disease that results from the interaction of both environmental and genetic factors (Bouchard, 1991). There is good evidence for a genetic component to human obesity, such as familial clustering (relative risk among sibs of 3–7) (Allison *et al.*, 1996) and the high concordance of body composition in monozygotic twins (Maes *et al.*, 1997). However, the role of genetic factors in common obesity is complex, being determined by the interaction of several genes (polygenic). Each of these may have relatively small effects (i.e. they are susceptibility genes) working in combination with each other as well as with environmental factors (such as nutrient intake, physical activity and smoking). As complex traits arise through the concerted action of multiple genetic influences and a variety of powerful environmental factors, the task of identifying any single susceptibility factor is always a problem.

26   *Philippe Froguel*

Monogenic forms of human obesity

Despite early evidence that genes must contribute to the variation in body fat in man, no obesity gene was identified until the *ob* gene was discovered in mice (Zhang, 1994). Most of the obesity-related syndromes, such as Prader-Willi, Cohen, Alström and Bardet-Biedl have now been genetically mapped. Causative genes have only been identified in three distinct Bardet-Biedl syndrome (BBS) loci. BBS6 (Katsanis *et al.*, 2000; Slavotinek *et al.*, 2000) is caused by mutations in the MKKS gene which presents homologies with a bacterial chaperonin. Genes responsible for BBS2 (Nishimura *et al.*, 2001) and BBS4 (Mykytyn *et al.*, 2001) code for proteins with unknown function. The rarity of these mutations has made the search for the causative genes difficult.

The alternative strategy, used with considerable success, is to screen extremely obese human subjects for mutations in candidate genes selected on the basis of mouse genetic studies. However, this approach limits investigation to previously suspected genes. Nevertheless, the findings of mutations in these homologous genes underscore the role of the underlying pathways in energy homoeostasis. Although infrequent, the opportunity to cure certain patients of their genetically determined obese phenotype has important implications for the development of similar therapies for the commoner forms of obesity. Five different obesity genes have been found in only three years: those coding for leptin and its receptor, pro-opiomelanocortin (POMC), melanocortin receptor 4 (MC4R) and the proconvertase 1 enzyme (PC1) Clement *et al.*, 1998; Jackson *et al.*, 1997; Krude *et al.*, 1998; Montague *et al.*, 1997; Vaisse *et al.*, 1998; Yeo *et al.*, 1998). All the proteins encoded by these five genes are part of the same pathway regulating food intake (Figure 3.1). Interestingly, no genetic mutation involved in the other numerous pathways regulating energy intake has been found in cases of human obesity, suggesting that the leptin pathway may be the pre-eminent regulator of energy balance in humans – or it may reveal our ignorance of most of the complex network of proteins regulating body weight. Despite its initial success, human genetics may still only explain a minority of mendelian forms of obesity. Animal studies as well as new genomic approaches will probably contribute to the discovery of new candidate genes also playing a role in monogenic human obesity.

The human genes causing monofactorial obesity fall into two categories. The first includes the genes coding for leptin, leptin receptor and POMC. Mutations in these genes induce rare, recessive forms of obesity associated with multiple endocrine dysfunctions. Two kindreds with defects in the leptin gene have been reported with loss-of-function mutations (Montague *et al.*, 1997; Strobel *et al.*, 1998). Homozygous carriers exhibit a similar phenotype

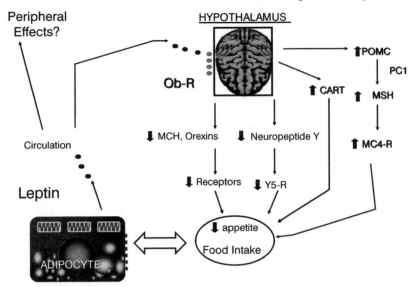

Figure 3.1 Leptin pathway for weight control. All the monogenic obesity gene-encoded proteins (Leptin, Ob-R, POMC, PC1, MC4R) are strongly connected as part of the same loop of regulation of food intake. Ob-R, leptin receptor gene; POMC, pro-opiomelanocortin; PCI, pro-hormone convertase-I; CART, cocaine and amphetamine-related transcript; α-MSH, α-melanocyte-stimulating hormone; MCH, melanin-concentrating hormone; MC4R, melanocortin-4 receptor. Reproduced by permission from *Best Practice and Research Clinical Endocrinology and Metabolism*, Vol. 15, No. 3 (in press).

of morbid obesity with onset in the first weeks of life, including severe hyperphagia, hypogonadotropic hypogonadism and central hypothyroidism. One family has been identified with a leptin receptor mutation (Clement *et al.*, 1998). In the three individuals with the homozygous mutation, a truncation of the receptor before the transmembrane domain completely abolished leptin signalling, leading to a phenotype similar to that of individuals with leptin deficiency, although more severe. The three sisters bearing the leptin receptor mutation also displayed significant growth retardation due to impaired growth hormone secretion. These obese subjects, as well as their heterozygous healthy parents, presented with very high levels of leptin. Chromatography of the circulating leptin revealed that the hormone was bound to the truncated leptin receptor, leading to increased plasma leptin half-life, although fat leptin expression remained correlated to the fat mass. The full knock-out of the leptin pathway in humans is not responsible for compensatory hypersecretion of leptin. Interestingly, the two girls bearing the mutation, who are still alive, are neither diabetic nor hyperlipidaemic.

The key role of the melanocortin system in the control of human body weight is evidenced by the discovery of mutations in the POMC and MC4R genes that also result in severe obesity. The POMC gene, expressed in human brain, gut, placenta and pancreas is involved in the leptin/melanocortin pathway (O'Donohue and Dorsa, 1982). Furthermore, POMC is the precursor of other peptides which include adrenocorticotropin (ACTH) and melanocyte-stimulating hormones (MSH) involved in energy homoeostasis (Woods *et al.*, 1998). POMC-knockout mice (Yaswen *et al.*, 1999) have obesity, defective adrenal development and altered pigmentation. These are similar to the phenotypes of patients with mutations in the coding region of the POMC gene (Krude *et al.*, 1998). Indeed, two children with homozygous or compound heterozygous loss-of-function mutations in POMC exhibited a phenotype reflecting the lack of pituitary neuropeptides derived from the POMC gene (Krude *et al.*, 1998). The absence of α-MSH was responsible for the ensuing obesity (as a result of the absence of the melanocortin ligand for MC4R) and altered pigmentation and red hair (resulting from the absence of the ligand for MC1R). The absence of ACTH led to adrenal deficiency through MC2R signal deficiency.

The second group of monogenic forms of obesity is related to non-syndromic obesity resulting from numerous mutations in the MC4R gene (Vaisse *et al.*, 1998; Vaisse *et al.*, 2000; Yeo *et al.*, 1998). The MC4R gene is the most prevalent obesity gene to date, being involved in 1–4 per cent of obese people (Vaisse *et al.*, 2000). MC4R mutations generally segregate in families under an autosomal dominant mode of inheritance with variable penetrance. In some consanguinous pedigrees, MC4R mutations with relatively modest loss of function appear to be co-dominantly or even recessively associated with obesity. The MC4R-associated human obesity phenotypes are similar to those found in mice lacking MC4R. These rodents show moderate to severe co-dominant obesity, more severe in homozygous than in heterozygous knock-out (KO) mice. The neuroendocrine function with regard to adrenals, growth, reproduction and thyroid is not altered. Human obesity caused by MC4R mutations is similar to more common forms of obesity, with an earlier age of onset and with a trend for hyperphagia in infancy, a trait that seems to disappear with age. Recent data obtained in mice as well as in humans suggest that impaired MC4R signalling could be involved in hyperinsulinaemia through impaired negative neuronal control of insulin secretion (Cone, 2000). In this respect, MC4R might be considered as a 'thrifty gene' (i.e. a gene whose product promotes energy efficiency) and could serve as a primary target for small anti-obesity molecules, regardless of the proximate cause of the obesity, and possibly as a target for drugs treating the metabolic syndrome (Vaisse *et al.*, 2000).

Genomic approach to common human obesity

Candidate gene studies

The common forms of obesity are polygenic. To date, most of the genes investigated have failed to give convincing and unambiguous evidence of their involvement in the genetic risk for obesity. Reasons are numerous, but include a lack of well-conducted studies of candidate genes in large populations with reliable phenotypes.

Two general approaches are used in the search for genes underlying common polygenic obesity in humans. The first one focuses on candidate genes, that is, genes having some plausible role in obesity, based on their known or presumed biological role in energy homeostasis. Efforts to identify candidate genes for obesity first concentrated on adipose tissue. In brown adipose tissue, regulation of thermogenesis by the sympathetic nervous system is mediated by β-adrenergic receptors (Nonogaki, 2000). In humans, the β_3-adrenergic receptors (β_3-AR) are modestly expressed in fat and adipocytes lining the gastrointestinal tract (Krief *et al.*, 1993). A Trp64Arg mutation located in the first trans-membrane domain of the receptor has been found to correlate with obesity, weight gain and insulin resistance in Pima Indians, the French and Finns (Clement *et al.*, 1995; Walston *et al.*, 1995; Widen *et al.*, 1995). Discordant associations as well as functional studies have also been published (Buettner *et al.*, 1998; Ghosh *et al.*, 1999), indicating that the role of this candidate gene in human obesity, if any, is modest, or should be considered in combination with other factors of the same pathway. In mature brown adipocyte cells, stimulation of β_3-AR by norepinephrine activates uncoupling protein 1 (UCP-1) via the cAMP metabolic pathway. Uncoupling proteins (UCPs) are inner mitochondrial membrane transporters that dissipate the proton gradient, releasing stored energy in the form of heat (Klingenberger, 1990). An A → G variation in UCP1 at position -3826 was associated with a gain of fat mass in a Quebec family study (Oppert *et al.*, 1994). Additional effects of the G allele of the A → G variant of UCP1 with the Trp64Arg mutation of the β_3-AR gene were found to occur in a morbidly obese French population (Clement *et al.*, 1996). Synergic effects of UCP1 with β_3-AR polymorphism in decreasing sympathetic nervous system activity was also observed in a Japanese population (Shihara *et al.*, 2001). Polymorphisms in other members of the uncoupling gene families, UCP2 and UCP3, correlated with body maas index in Pima Indians (Walder *et al.*, 1998). A common polymorphism in the promoter of UCP2 is associated with enhanced mRNA expression and decreased risk of obesity (Esterbauer *et al.*, 2001), while no effect was described with other genetic variations in Caucasians (Otabe *et al.*, 1998). Recent data from UCP2 KO mice

(Arsenijevic *et al.*, 2001) showed no effect on body weight, but they were nevertheless hyperinsulinaemic. Further studies showed that UCP2 is a potent inhibitor of insulin secretion (Zhang *et al.*, 2001).

All these uncertainties illustrate the complexity of the candidate gene approach, especially when gene function is not completely understood. Interaction studies between the genetic variation in candidate genes and environmental factors need to be explored. For example, a polymorphism in the UCP3 gene was shown to modify the benefit of physical activity on body weight (Otabe *et al.*, 2000). The role of physical activity in the relationships between the phenotypic expression of obesity and a genetic variation in the β_2-adrenergic receptor has also been described in a French male cohort (Meirhaeghe *et al.*, 1999).

As frequently reported, the candidate gene approach has, thus far, only yielded likely susceptibility genes with a small or uncertain effects (Barsh *et al.*, 2000, Perusse *et al.*, 2001). Extensive gene targeting experiments in mice, together with functional genomics (expression profiles in different tissues of interest for energy balance), together with the near-completion of the Human Genome Project, provide a new generation of candidate genes for obesity. The choice of an ideal candidate gene may be based on several criteria including, but not limited to:

•   Chromosomal localization near an obesity-linked locus in human or in animal models.
•   Expression profile (i.e. in adipocyte or in hypothalamus).
•   Expression regulated by food intake, nutrients or by physical activity.
•   Gene targeting or overexpression modifying body weight.

Genome-wide scans for obesity

The second approach to identifying genes underlying common polygenic obesity utilizes genome-wide scans in order to detect chromosomal regions showing linkage with obesity in large collections of nuclear families. This strategy makes no presumption as to the function of genes at the susceptibility loci, since it attempts to map genes purely by position. Identification of such susceptibility gene(s) for obesity may then be positionally cloned in the intervals of linkage.

Five genome-wide scans for obesity genes have been published to date. These were carried out in Mexican American families (Comuzzie *et al.*, 1997), French pedigrees (Hager *et al.*, 1998), Pima Indians (Hanson *et al.*, 1998; Norman *et al.*, 1997), White Americans (Kissebah *et al.*, 2000; Lee *et al.*, 1999) and in the Amish (Hsueh *et al.*, 2001). Both Comuzzie *et al.*, (1997) and Hager *et al.*, (1998) provided a candidate region on chromosome 2p21 that could explain a significant part of the variance of leptin levels in humans. This linkage was replicated in a cohort of African American families (Rotimi *et al.*, 1999). Other major genetic loci for obesity and leptin levels (Figure 3.2) were identified on chromosome 10p11 and on 5cen-q in French families. This 10p locus may account for 20–30 per cent of the genetic risk for obesity in this population (Hager *et al.*, 1998), and was recently confirmed in a cohort of obese German youths (Hinney *et al.*, 2000), as well as in white Caucasians, African Americans (Price *et al.*, 2001), and in the in-bred Amish (Hsueh *et al.*, 2001). In addition to this 10p locus, a genome scan performed in white Americans showed evidence for linkage on chromosome 20q 13 and on 10q (Lee *et al.*, 1999). In Pima Indians the most interesting region was shown on chromosome 11q (Norman *et al.*, 1997). Comuzzie *et al.* also described a new locus at 3q27 which was linked to various quantitative traits characterizing the metabolic/insulin resistance syndrome (Kissebah *et al.*, 2000), a locus previously identified as a T2DM locus in the French population (Vionnet *et al.*, 2000). Several candidate genes map to this region, including the APM1 gene encoding the differentiated adipocyte secreted protein ACRP30/adiponectin, which is abundantly present in the plasma. The purified C-terminal domain of adiponectin has been reported to protect mice on a high-fat diet from obesity. It rescued obese or lipoatropic mice models from severe insulin resistance, by decreasing levels of plasma free fatty acids (FFA) and enhancing lipid oxidization in muscle (Fruebis *et al.*, 2001). Plasma levels of adiponectin were shown to be decreased in obese diabetic subjects (Arita *et al.*, 1999). Decreased adiponectin is implicated in the development of insulin resistance in mouse models of both obesity and lipoatrophy (Yamauchi *et al.*, 2001), which makes ACRP30 an attractive candidate gene for fat-induced metabolic syndrome and type 2 diabetes mellitus. Further studies will address the role of variations in the ACRP30 gene in obesity or in obesity-associated type 2 diabetes.

Some concerns, mostly regarding lack of replication, have been raised about the heterogeneity and reliability of genetic data in multifactorial diseases in general. The results from genome scans in obesity studies are surprisingly reproducible, despite differences in ethnicity and in environmental factors. Indeed, loci on chromosomes 2 and 10 are largely confirmed, as well as, to a lesser extent, loci on chromosome 5. These data suggest that a few major loci may contribute to the genetic risk for obesity and related phenotypes in humans. A working hypothesis based on available data is that obesity is an oligogenic disease whose development can be modulated by various polygenic (modifier genes) and environmental influences. The challenge is now to identify the true aetiological gene variants, explaining these genome-wide scan results.

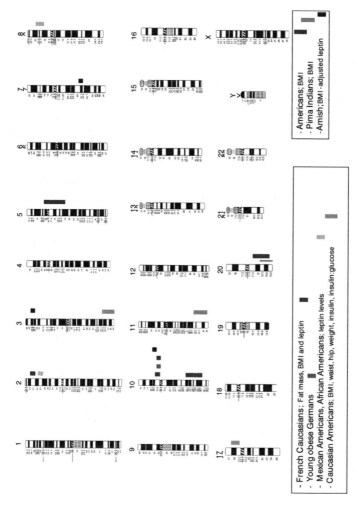

Figure 3.2 Chromosomal location of obesity loci identified in genome-wide scan studies. Reproduced by permission from *Best Practice and Research Clinical Endocrinology and Metabolism*, Vol. 15, No. 3 (in press).

Positional cloning strategy

To be identified with an enhanced risk for overweight, chromosomal regions of linkage should be firstly be refined using a dense map of biallelic single-nucleotide polymorphisms (SNPs). The state of the art in positional cloning of complex disorder susceptibility genes involves the systematic use of SNP markers for the detection of linkage disequilibrium (LD) mapping (Abecasis *et al.*, 2001; Terwilliger and Weiss, 1998). DNA polymorphisms located away from the true functional variant can be associated with the trait or with a variation of an obesity-associated trait. The strength of LD is variable within the genome, ranging from 10 kb to 300 kb or more. It was postulated that working in so-called 'isolated' populations would significantly increase LD expectancy, but recent evidence from work in Finns and Icelanders shows that this is not the case (Eaves *et al.*, 2000). The recent identification of the NIDDM1 gene (calpain 10) on 2q confirmed that LD mapping could be a successful strategy to unravel other polygenic diseases (Horikawa *et al.*, 2000). This work also showed the complexity of the search. In this case, an intronic polymorphism (UCSNP-43) was associated with type 2 diabetes in Mexican Americans. In fact, three non-coding polymorphisms, including UCSNP-43, have been identified, defining an at-risk haplotype. In other ethnic groups, such as French Caucasians, the rarity of this high-risk haplotype makes it difficult to provide a definite answer about the role of calpain 10 in type 2 diabetes. Moreover, as the function of this protease is still unclear, this study has emphasized the limitation of genetic studies in proving a functional relation from methods based solely on statistics.

To be efficient, LD mapping should be integrated with both genetic and functional studies. For example, tissue profiling may provide the most direct way of improving overall understanding of the molecular circuitry maintaining energy homoeostasis. Therefore, expression profiling in humans on the one hand, and genetic analysis of populations on the other, will provide complementary tools to advance our understanding of the complex network of gene–gene and gene–environment interactions underlying the susceptibility to obesity. Following identification of genetic variations, exploration of the consequences at tissue level (tissue profiling), the organism and the population level (molecular epidemiology) will clarify the role of these variants in the disease pathogenesis and their implications for diagnostic and therapeutic developments. Improved understanding of genetic and environmental predictors of risk factors provides a rational basis for stratification of the disease risk and the response to treatment, allowing effective targeting of preventive and therapeutic tools.

34   *Philippe Froguel*

Conclusion

The current epidemic of obesity presents a major public health challenge, given the strong association of adiposity with cardiovascular, metabolic and other diseases. Preventive and therapeutic approaches are hampered by a lack of fundamental understanding of the control of human body fat mass and disturbance of this control in obese states. Human geneticists have pioneered the understanding of the genetic basis of obesity through their discovery of the first monogenic defects leading to extreme childhood obesity. The more challenging problem is identification of the genetic variants which underlie susceptibility to the common forms of human obesity. Given high-quality family material and recently confirmed genome-wide scan results, it is likely that aetiological variants in candidate genes will emerge. The success of these studies will require a multidisciplinary approach combining genomics, bioinformatics, expression profiling, biochemistry, human physiology and molecular epidemiology. While the task is considerable, the breadth and depth of expertise now available in the genetics of complex human traits provide unique scientific opportunities for significant advances.

References

Abecasis, G.R., Noguchi, E., Heinzmann, A. *et al.* (2000) Extent and distribution of linkage disequilibrium in three genomic regions. *Am J Hum Genet*, 68:191–7.

Allison, D.B., Faith, M.S. and Nathan, J.S. (1996) Risch's lambda values for human obesity. *Int J Obes*, 20: 990–9.

Arita, Y., Kihara, S. *et al.* (1999) Paradoxical decrease of an adipose-specific protein, adiponectin, in obesity. *Biochem Biophys Res Commun*, 257: 79–83.

Arsenijevic, D., Numa, H., Pecqueur, C. *et al.* (2000) Disruption of the uncoupling protein-2 gene in mice reveals a role in immunity reactive oxygen species production. *Nature Genet*, 26: 435–9.

Barsh, G.S., Farooqi, I.S. and O'Rahilly, S. (2000) Genetics of body-weight regulation. *Nature*, 404: 644–51.

Bouchard, C. (1991) Current understanding of aetiology of obesity genetic and non genetic factors. *Am J Clin Nutr*, 53: 1561–5.

Buettner, R., Schaffler, R.D., Arndt, H. *et al.* (1998) The Trp64Arg polymorphism of the beta3-adrenergic receptor gene is not associated with obesity or type 2 diabetes mellitus in a large population-based caucasian cohort. *J Clin Endocrinol Metab*, 83(11): 2892–7.

Clement, K., Ruiz, J., Cassard-Doulcier, A.M. *et al.* (1996) Additive effects of polymorphisms in the uncoupling protein gene and the beta3-adrenergic receptor gene on weight gain in morbid obesity. *Int J Obes*, 20: 1062–6.

Clement, K., Vaisse, C., Lahlou, N. *et al.* (1998) A mutation in the human leptin receptor gene causes obesity and pituitary dysfunction. *Nature*, 392: 398–401.

Clement, K., Vaisse, C., Manning, B.S.J. *et al.* (1995) Genetic variation in the beta3-adrenergic receptor gene and an increased capacity to gain weight in patients with morbid obesity. *N Engl J Med*, 333: 352–4.

Comuzzie, A.G., Hixson, J.E., Almasy, L. *et al.* (1997) A major quantitative trait locus determining serum leptin levels and fat mass is located on human chromosome 2. *Nature Genet*, 15: 273–6.

Cone, R.D. (2000) Haploinsufficiency of the melanocortin-4 receptor deficiency. *J Clin Invest*, 106: 185–7.

Eaves, I.A., Merriman, T.R., Barber, R.A. *et al.* (2000) The genetically isolated populations of Finland and Sardinia may not be a panacea for linkage disequilibrium mapping of common disease genes. *Nature Genet*, 25: 320–3.

Esterbauer, D., Schneitler, C., Oberkofler, H. *et al.* (2001) A common polymorphism in the promoter of UCP2 is associated with decreased risk of obesity in middle-aged humans. *Nature Genet*, 28: 178–83.

Farooqi, S., Jebb, S., Langmak, G. *et al.* (1999) Effects of recombinant leptin therapy in a child with congenital leptin deficiency. *N Engl J Med*, 341: 879–84.

Fruebis, J., Tsao, T., Javorschi, S. *et al.* (2001) Proteolytic cleavage product of 30-kDa adipocyte complement-related protein increases fatty acid oxidation in muscle and causes weight loss in mice. *Proc Natl Acad Sci USA*, 98: 2005–10.

Ghosh, S., Langefeld, C.D., Ally, D. *et al.* (1999) The W64R variant of the beta3-adrenergic receptor gene is not associated with type 2 diabetes or obesity in a large Finnish sample. *Diabetologia*, 42(2): 238–44.

Hager, J., Dina, C., Francke, S. *et al.* (1998) A genome-wide scan for human obesity genes shows evidence for a major susceptibility locus on chromosome 10. *Nature Genet*, 20: 304–38.

Hanson, R.L., Ehm, M.G., Pettitt, D.J. *et al.* (1998) An autosomal genomic scan for loci linked to type II diabetes mellitus and body-mass index in Pima indians. *Am J Hum Genet*, 63: 1130–8.

Hinney, A., Ziegler, A., Oeffner, F. *et al.* (2000) Independent confirmation of a major locus for obesity on chromosome 10. *J Clin Endocrinol Metab*, 85: 2962–5.

Horikawa, Y., Oda, N., Cox, N.J. *et al.* (2000) Genetic variation in the gene encoding calpain-10 is associated with type 2 diabetes mellitus. *Nature Genet*, 26: 163–75.

Hsueh, W.C., Mitchell, B.D., Schneider, J.L. *et al.* (2001) Genome-wide scan of obesity in the old order Amish. *J Clin Endocrinol Metab*, 86: 1199–205.

Jackson, R.S., Creemers, J.W., Ohagi, S. *et al.* (1997) Obesity and impaired pro-hormone processing associated with mutations in the human prohormone convertase 1 gene. *Nature Genet*, 16: 303–6.

Katsanis, N., Beales, P.L., Woods, M.O. *et al.* (2000) Mutations in MKKS cause obesity, retinal dystrophy and renal malformations associated with Bardet-Biedl syndrome. *Nature Genet*, 26: 67–70.

Kissebah, A.H., Sonnenberg, G.E., Myklebust, J. *et al.* (2000) Quantitative trait loci on chromosome 3 and 17 influence phenotypes of the metabolic syndrome. *Proc Natl Acad Sci USA*, 97: 14478–83.

Klingenberger, M. (1990) Mechanism and evolution of the uncoupling protein of brown adipose tissue. *Trends Biochem Sci*, 15: 108–12.

Krief, S., Lonnqvist, F., Raimbault, S., *et al.* (1993) Tissue distribution of β_3-adrenergic receptor nRNA in man. *J Clin Invest*, 91: 344–9.

Krude, H., Biebermann, H., Luck, W. *et al.* (1998) A severe early-onset obesity, adrenal insufficiency and red hair pigmentation caused by POMC mutations in humans. *Nature Genet*, 19: 155–7.

Lean, M.E.J., Hans, T.S. and Seidell, J.C. (1998) Impairment of health and quality of life in people with large waist circumference. *Lancet*, 351: 853–6.

Lee, J.H., Reed, D.R., Li, W.D. *et al.* (1999) Genome scan for human obesity and linkage to markers in 20q13. *Am J Hum Genet*, 64: 196–209.

Maes, H.H., Neale, M.C. and Eaves, L.J. (1997) Genetic and environmental factors in relative body weight and human adiposity. *Behavior Genet*, 27: 325–51.

Maillard, G., Charles, M.A., Tibult, N. *et al.* (2000) Trends in the prevalence of obesity in children and adolescents in France between 1980 and 1991. *Int J Obesity*, 24(12): 1608–17.

Meirhaeghe, A., Helbecque, N., Cottel, D. and Amouyel, P. (1999) β_2-adrenoceptor gene polymorphism, body weight and physical activity. *Lancet*, 13: 896.

Montague, C.T., Farooqi, I.S., Whitehead, J.P. *et al.* (1997) Congenital leptin deficiency is associated with severe early-onset obesity in humans. *Nature*, 387: 903–8.

Mykytyn, K., Braun, T., Carmi, R. *et al.* (2001) Identification of the gene that, when mutated, causes the human obesity syndrome BBS4. *Nature Genet*, 28: 188–91.

Nishimura, D.Y. *et al.* (2001) Positional cloning of a novel gene on chromosome 16q causing Bardet-Biedl syndrome (BBS2). *Hum Mol Genet*, 10: 865–74.

Nonogaki, K. (2000) New insights into sympathetic regulation of glucose and fat metabolism. *Diabetologia*, 43: 533–49.

Norman, R.A., Thompson, D.B., Foroud, T. *et al.* (1997) Genomewide search for genes influencing percent body fat in Pima Indians: suggestive linkage at chromosome 11q21-q22. *Am J Hum Genet*, 60: 166–73.

O'Donohue, T.L. and Dorsa, D.M. (1982) The opiomelanotropinergic neuronal and endocrine systems. *Peptides*, 3: 353–95.

Oppert, J.M., Vohl, M.C., Chagnon, Y.C. *et al.* (1994) DNA polymorphism in the uncoupling protein (UCP) gene and human body fat. *Int J Obes*, 18: 526–31.

Otabe, S., Clement, K., Dina, C. *et al.* (2000) A genetic variation in the 5′ flanking region of the UCP3 gene is asociated with body mass index in humans in interaction with physical activity. *Diabetologia*, 43(2): 245–9.

Otabe, S., Clement, K., Rich, N. *et al.* (1998) Mutation screening of the human UCP2 gene in normoglycemic and NIDDM morbidly obese patients. *Diabetes*, 47: 840–2.

Perusse, L., Chagnon, Y.C., Weisnagel, S.J. *et al.* (2001) The human obesity gene map: the 2000 update. *Obesity Res*, 9: 135–69.

Prescott-Clarke, P. and Primatesta, P. (1998) *Health Survey for England 1996*. London: The Stationery Office.

Price, R.A., Li, W.D., Bernstein, A., Crystal, A. *et al.* (2001) A locus affecting obesity in human chromosome region 10p12. *Diabetologia*, 44: 363–6.

Rotimi, C.N., Comuzzie, A.G., Lowe, W.L. *et al.* (1999) The quantitative trait locus on chromosome 2 for serum leptin levels is confirmed in African-Americans. *Diabetes*, 48: 643–4.

Shihara, N., Yasuda, K., Moritani, T. *et al.* (2001) Synergic effect of polymorphisms of uncoupling protein1 and beta3-adrenergic receptor genes on autonomic nervous system activity. *Int J Obes Relat Metab Disord*, 25(6): 761–6.

Slavotinek, A.M., Stone, E.M., Mykytyn, K. *et al.* (2000) Mutations in MKKS cause Bardet-Biedl syndrome. *Nature Genet*, 26: 15–16.

Strobel, A., Issad, T., Camoin, L., Ozata, M. and Strosberg, A.D. (1998) A leptin missense mutation associated with hypogonadism and morbid obesity. *Nature Genet*, 18: 213–15.

Terwilliger, J.D. and Weiss, K.M. (1998) Linkage disequilibrium mapping of complex disease: fantasy or reality? *Curr Opin Biotechnol*, 9: 578–94.

Vaisse, C., Clement, K., Durand, E. *et al.* (2000) Melanocortin-4 receptor mutations are a frequent and heterogeneous cause of morbid obesity. *J Clin Invest*, 106: 253–62.

Vaisse, C., Clement, K., Guy, G.B. and Froguel, P. (1998) A frameshift mutation in human MC4R is associated with a dominant form of obesity. *Nature Genet*, 20: 113–14

Vionnet, N., Hani, E.H., Dupont, S. *et al.* (2000) Genomewide search for type 2 diabetes-susceptibility genes in French whites: evidence for a novel susceptibility locus for early-onset diabetes on chromosome 3q27-qter and independent replication of a type 2-diabetes locus on chromosome 1q21-q24. *Am J Hum Genet*, 67: 1470–80.

Walder, K., Norman, R., Hanson, R.L. *et al.* (1998) Association between uncoupling protein polymorphisms (UCP2-UCP3) and energy metabolism obesity in Pima Indians. *Hum Mol Genet*, 7: 1431–5.

Walston, J., Silver, K., Bogardus, C. *et al.* (1995) Time of onset of non-insulin dependent diabetes mellitus and genetic variation in the beta3-adrenergic receptor gene. *N Engl J Med*, 333: 343–8.

Widen, E., Lehto, M., Kanninen, T. *et al.* (1995) Association of a polymorphism in the β_3-adrenergic receptor gene with features of the insulin resistance syndrome in Finns. *N Engl J Med*, 333: 348–52.

Woods, S.C., Seeley, R.J., Porte, D. *et al.* (1998) Signals that regulate food intake and energy homeostasis. *Science*, 280: 1378–83.

World Health Organization (1997) *Obesity: Preventing and Managing the Global Epidemic.* Report of a WHO consultation on obesity. World Health Organization, Geneva, 3–5 June.

Yamauchi, T., Kamon, J., Waki, H. *et al.* (2001) The fat-derived hormone adiponectin reverses insulin resistance associated with both lipoatrophy and obesity. *Nature Med*, 7: 941–6.

Yaswen, L., Diehl, N., Brennan, M.B. and Hochgeschwender, U. (1999) Obesity in the mouse model of proopiomelanocortin deficiency responds to peripheral melanocortin. *Nature Med*, 5: 1066–70.

Yeo, G.S., Farooqi, I.S., Aminian, S. *et al.* (1998) A frameshift mutation in MC4R associated with dominantly inherited human obesity. *Nature Genet*, 20: 111–12.

Zhang, C.Y., Baffy, G., Perret, P. *et al.* (2001) Uncoupling protein-2 negatively regulates insulin secretion and is a major link between obesity, beta cell dysfunction, and type 2 diabetes. *Cell*, 15(6): 745–55.

Zhang, Y. (1994) Positional cloning of the mouse obese gene and its human homologue. *Nature*, 372: 425–32.

Zollner, S. and Von Haeseler, A. (2000) A coalescent approach to study linkage disequilibrium between single-nucleotide polymorphisms. *Am J Hum Genet*, 66: 615–28.

4 The seeds are sown in childhood

Terry Wilkin

Earlier chapters in this book have covered the global nature of obesity, the relationship between physical activity and food intake and some exciting developments in the genetics of obesity. This chapter will try to link obesity with some of the problems that result from it by exploring the underlying mechanisms that affect health. In the case of obesity, the underlying process is that of insulin resistance. This chapter will ask four questions and conclude with four challenges.

What is insulin resistance?

To understand insulin resistance, it is first necessary to define control and explore the operation of a negative feedback control loop. Control is the process responsible for maintaining the concentration of a substance within tight limits. It is a mechanism of constraint, and fundamental to health (Wilkin, 1998). The negative feedback loop responsible for maintaining, for example, the concentration of blood glucose within healthy limits uses insulin from the pancreatic islets to control the flux of glucose across the tissues – principally liver, fat and muscle. Insufficient insulin permits the blood glucose concentration to rise. As there are only two components to all control loops, there are essentially only two ways in which the glucose loop can go wrong. Either the islets fail, or the tissues fail.

Failure of the islets leads to type 1 diabetes. By definition, type 1 diabetes is a state of high blood glucose and low blood insulin. The process is conceptually straightforward: gradual loss of islets, loss of insulin and a rise in blood glucose. Islet cell destruction may take place slowly over a period of months or years – the duration can vary considerably – but destruction of the islets leads, inexorably, to the rise in blood glucose. Failure of the tissues, on the other hand, results in a quite different situation. By 'failure of the tissues' is meant a loss of their responsiveness to insulin – so-called insulin resistance. Insulin resistance most commonly results from weight gain and physical inactivity, and is the process that leads to type 2 diabetes. As tissue resistance to insulin rises, so the islets release more insulin, but their capacity is ultimately exhausted, at which point the blood sugar also rises. In contrast to type 1 diabetes, the process leading to type 2 is characterized by high glucose *and* high insulin levels. It is this rise in blood insulin that disturbs the metabolic systems which are associated with cardiovascular risk.

If the clinical event is the explosion, insulin resistance is the fuse that precedes it. The prevention of diabetes will require a detailed understanding of what ignites the fuse, what fuels it and, most importantly, how best to extinguish it before the explosion occurs. The first key message, therefore, is that type 2 diabetes is the *outcome* of a process, it is not the process itself. The process is one of insulin resistance.

What are the effects of insulin resistance?

Hyperglycaemia leading to diabetes is one effect of insulin resistance. Hyperglycaemia is serious in the long term because of the microvascular changes caused by tissue glycosylation, but it is not as serious as the hyperinsulinaemia that causes macrovascular disease by accelerating atherosclerosis. Provided that the beta cells respond with sufficient insulin to meet the resistance, the situation may remain one of 'silent' hyperinsulinaemia characterized by 'high normal', but not overtly diabetic, blood glucose levels for many years. High insulin levels, however, disturb blood lipids, and lead to hyperlipidaemia. There are also disturbances in blood pressure, packed cell volume, coagulation factors produced by the liver and in uric acid levels, leading to hypertension, hyperviscosity, hypercoaguability and hyperuricemia. Each is a cardiovascular risk factor in its own right, but deadly in combination (Bonora *et al.*, 1998). High blood sugars seldom kill in type 2 diabetes. Death is most commonly cardiovascular. It is only in the last 15 years, since Reaven first linked insulin resistance with cardiovascular risk in the so-called 'syndrome X' or 'metabolic syndrome', that these relationships have become clearer (Reaven, 1988). The six metabolic disturbances resulting from hyperinsulinaemia are popularly referred to as the 'deadly sextet' (Enzi *et al.*, 1993).

The metabolic syndrome can be viewed as a cartwheel, with insulin resistance as the hub. There are six spokes (the sextet), each in its own right an independent risk factor for early cardiovascular death, but in combination responsible for the premature mortality attributable to vascular disease which has characterized the past 50 years in industrialized societies. Recently, it has become clear that there is a seventh spoke, not a killer in the same way, but nevertheless an important condition in daily clinical practice. Clinicians had long been aware of a syndrome associated with overweight, hirsutism, amenorrhoea and infertility, but were unsure as to its cause. For many years it was known as Stein-Leventhal syndrome, more recently as polycystic ovary syndrome (PCOS) (Franks, 1995). This has turned out to be yet another effect of high insulin levels, this time driving the thecal cells of the ovary to produce excess amounts of testosterone. It is the resulting imbalance between testosterone and oestrogen that leads to the clinical signs and symptoms. Like the other spokes on the wheel, PCOS will improve by reducing insulin resistance. PCOS is, predictably, a strong marker for future diabetes. New insights into pre-eclamptic toxaemia suggest that it may be set to become an eighth spoke (Kaaja *et al.*, 1999).

The second message, accordingly, is that diabetes is not a disease in isolation. It is part of a broader metabolic disorder – a syndrome that kills prematurely – with insulin resistance playing a key role. Indeed, type 2 diabetes is not primarily a disorder of glucose metabolism. It is primarily a disorder of lipid metabolism.

What causes insulin resistance?

Some 50 years ago, a Frenchman by the name of Jean Vague commented on two distributions of body fat, the one subcutaneous and the other visceral or intra-abdominal (Vague, 1956). He referred to obese people as either *pommes* (apples) or *poires* (pears), according to differences in body shape. He also made the seminal observation that obese people whose excess fat mass was carried high in the abdomen (the 'apples') were at greater cardiovascular risk than the those of the same weight who carried it lower down. Most such 'pears' are female. Oestrogen tends to drive fat down into the gluteofemoral regions where fat is subcutaneous. Fat in this location has few metabolic implications. 'Apples', on the other hand, are most often though – not exclusively – male, because testosterone drives fat into the abdomen.

Visceral fat is contained within the cavity of the abdomen, not under the skin. It can be seen clearly in Figure 4.1. Unlike subcutaneous fat, the free fatty acids produced by visceral fat pass directly to the liver, where they influence insulin resistance. A strong correlation has been shown between the percentage of abdominal fat and insulin resistance across the range of body mass index (BMI; Figure 4.2; Carey *et al.*, 1996). In another study (Zavaroni, 1989), Italian factory workers were divided into two groups according to high or average insulin resistance, but were matched for age and BMI (Table 4.1). One hour after a glucose load, the insulin levels in the resistant group were significantly higher, as were their blood pressure, glucose, triglyceride and cholesterol levels. As the groups were matched for BMI, the study demonstrates vividly how insulin resistance is more important to metabolic health than BMI which says nothing about fat distribution. It is of interest in this regard that sumo wrestlers, sometimes weighing more

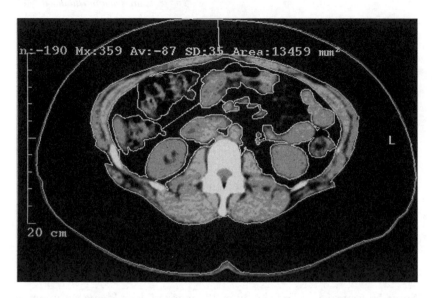

Figure 4.1 A CT scan of the abdomen in an obese female. The black areas denote fat. Although there is a considerable amount of intra-abdominal (visceral) fat, there is yet more located subcutaneously.

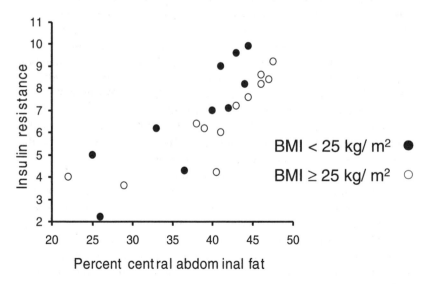

Figure 4.2 The relationship between intra-abdominal (visceral) fat and insulin resistance. BMI is not a good indicator of insulin resistance as those of high and low BMI are indistinguishable in this relationship.

Table 4.1 A summary of the data from Zavaroni's study of Italian factory workers

	Insulin resistance	
	Normal	*High*
Age	39	39
BMI	24.7	24.7
Insulin, 1h (ml/l)	35	94*
Glucose, 1h (mg/dl)	94	110*
Triglycerides (mmol/l	1.2	1.7*
Cholesterol (mmol/l)	4.8	5.1*
BP systolic (mm Hg)	119	126*
BP diastolic (mm Hg)	78	85*

Note: * p <0.005. When divided up according to insulin resistance, but matched for BMI, the disturbances which characterize the metabolic syndrome were more advanced in those with the higher intra-abdominal fat content.

Source: Adapted from Zavaroni *et al.*, 1989

than 200 kg, are not insulin resistant because the greater proportion of the fat measured in their girth is deposited subcutaneously, and not within the abdominal cavity (Matsuzawa, 1997). This favourable distribution of body fat is achieved by intense physical training. However, sumo wrestlers acquire large amounts of visceral fat on retirement, when they cease to train, and they die prematurely from cardiovascular disease, often after many years of diabetes.

The biochemistry relating adipose tissue to insulin resistance is complex and not fully understood. Adipose tissue does not only produce free fatty acids, but hormonal-like substances which include fibronectin, resistin, leptin and TNF-α. These substances impact upon the liver and other tissues to induce insulin resistance. The liver is the first stop for a flux of free fatty acids and chylomicrons which, in turn, are the substrate for triglycerides. Triglyceride levels are consequently high in individuals with a high fat mass and are in themselves an independent risk factor for cardiovascular disease. There are further implications because a high concentration of triglycerides begins to distort unfavourably the ratios between the HDL and LDL cholesterols. The free fatty acids are also thought to compete for the utilization of glucose by muscle in the Randle cycle, rendering the muscle relatively insulin-resistant (Randle, 1966). Much detail has yet to be worked out, most intriguingly in relation to the hypothalamic–pituitary–adrenal (HPA) axis. Cushing's disease, characterized by disturbance of the HPA axis and hyper-cortisolaemia, is an unexpected model for metabolic syndrome, with abdominal obesity and insulin resistance as central features.

The third message, therefore – and an important one clinically – is that total fat is not the cause of insulin resistance. The distribution of that fat is the critical factor (Ruderman *et al.*, 1998; Montague and O'Rahilly, 2000). BMI is widely used as a measure of fatness. Importantly, however, it is not a measure of fat distribution.

When does insulin resistance begin?

Various hypotheses have asserted that insulin resistance may have early origins, either as a result of genetic inheritance or because of gestational programming. There are three principal theories – the *thrifty genotype hypothesis* (Neel, 1962), which argues for genetically programmed insulin over-production to which the body responds with anti-insulins (resistance), the *thrifty phenotype hypothesis* (Hales and Barker, 1992), which cites maternal malnutrition as the basis for fetal insulin resistance as an adaptive response, and the *fetal insulin hypothesis* (Hattersley and Tooke, 1999), which predicts the involvement of insulin resistance genes.

The thrifty phenotype hypothesis by Hales and Barker has enjoyed much the greatest exposure. The observations, initially made from a cohort born in Hertfordshire some 80 years ago, were that metabolic disturbances later in life correlated (inversely) with birth weight, and that low birth weight was associated with high insulin resistance in middle life. The assumption drawn from the associations was that birth weight reflects only pre-natal events. The hypothesis argues that pre-natal events responsible for low birth weight (and malnutrition would, of course, be a key event) are also responsible for the insulin resistance that has its impact later in life. There have been a number of challenges to this hypothesis. One concern is that birth weight is not necessarily a physiological surrogate for what goes on in gestation, but merely a statistical association. What happens *after* birth correlates as much with birth weight as what happens *before* birth. To implicate a pre-natal experience in the later outcome, using birth weight as a surrogate for that experience, is to overlook the possibility that there could be a more important post-natal factor correlating with birth weight. This is a statistical argument, first proposed by Lucas and colleagues (1999), but it is supported by clinical data from the EarlyBird Study currently under way in Plymouth.

The EarlyBird Study

EarlyBird is a prospective, non-intervention cohort study of 300 healthy children at school entry, and designed to answer the question: 'Which children develop insulin resistance, and why?' These children are reviewed every 6 months, when a number of anthropometric and metabolic investigations are carried out. Baseline data on the whole cohort is now complete, and has made some important findings. The first is neither unique nor complicated – that low birth weight in the UK is no longer a common occurrence. The initial studies carried out by Barker involved cohorts from an earlier era. Both the UK and Finnish cohorts, subsequently used to support the *thrifty phenotype hypothesis*, looked back to pre-Second World War births, when birth weights below 2,500 gms were more common (Forsen *et al.*, 2000). Low birth weight may well reflect a gestational process responsible for insulin resistance, but it is no longer a problem in the UK or, indeed, the westernized world. It is unlikely, therefore, that low birth weight, or whatever it represents in gestational terms, is responsible for the exponential rise in type 2 diabetes that we are currently witnessing.

The EarlyBird Study has measured insulin resistance levels in boys and girls at 5 years of age, but has found no relationship with birth weight in either sex. There is, however, a clear relationship between *current* weight and insulin resistance, particularly in the girls. The relationship between body mass and insulin resistance is stronger still in the mothers, pointing to an inevitable and inexorable rise in levels of insulin resistance as these children grow and mature. These data confirm the observation of Whincup and colleagues that current weight, rather than birth weight, appears to determine insulin resistance in contemporary children (Whincup *et al.*, 1997). While it is of concern that the process of insulin resistance can start so early in life, it is, at the same time, encouraging that the lifestyle factors threatening the health of today's children appear to be post-natal rather than pre-natal, because the former may be more easily modified.

A further component of the programming argument has been the notion of 'catch-up' weight. For paediatricians accustomed to using centile charts, the concept of 'catch-up' growth poses no particular difficulty. It implies the re-establishment of the growth trajectory after a period of physical or psychological ill health (Prader, 1978). It has been suggested that in addition to low birth weight, catch-up – that is to say the extent to which centiles are crossed from birth – is an independent and additional cause of insulin resistance (Cianfarani *et al.*, 1999). Baseline data on 5-year-old children from the EarlyBird Study find no evidence to support the catch-up hypothesis. We divided the children into two groups, those above and those below median weight at birth. We also divided them into those above or below the median weight at five years, thus producing four cells. One group was of relatively low birth weight and remained relatively low-weight at 5 years of age (*low–low*). Another group was relatively light at birth and relatively heavy at 5 years (*low–high*), that is, the catch-up group. The remaining two groups were those who had been relatively heavy at birth and remained heavy (*high–high*) and the so-called 'catch-down' group (*high–low*). First we examined whether children of relatively low birth weight who remained relatively light had lower levels of insulin resistance than those who had 'caught up'. In common with previous studies, we found that they did. What the other studies had not done, however, was to look at those who were never of low birth weight but had achieved the same weight at 5 as those who had caught up, that is, the *high–high* group. The question we asked was: 'Is insulin resistance at 5 years of age determined by the weight you reach by 5, or the weight you started from at birth?' When we compared the *low–high* and the *high–high* groups, we found no difference. Insulin resistance in the catch-ups was no higher than in those who had been heavy all the time.

We are therefore cautious about interpreting 'catch-up growth' as something physiologically different from merely achieving a particular weight at 5 years. Indeed, when we examined the relationship between weight at five and change in weight since birth, in other words *catch-up* against *current* weight, we found a very close correlation, suggesting they are co-correlates, not independent factors. Those children who are heaviest now are merely those who have crossed the most centile lines. In a multiple regression analysis, the addition of catch-up to the relationship between weight or BMI at 5 and insulin resistance added nothing to the prediction. The data suggest that insulin resistance in contemporary UK children is not associated with birth weight, nor is it associated with catch-up weight. It is related to current weight. This message is important because a characteristic that is pro-grammed may be difficult to alter, whereas one acquired after birth is potentially modifiable.

Physical activity is undoubtedly a key factor in the development of child-hood obesity, as suggested by further, preliminary data from the EarlyBird Study where each child has worn a physical activity monitor, during waking hours, for 7-day periods. These accelerometers are smaller than a matchbox, unobtrusive and well tolerated. They provide a window on physical activity that we never had access to before, by allowing the timing, duration and intensity of activity to be recorded, second by second, over a period of days (Figure 4.3). The data show, first, an almost threefold difference between the most active and least active child. Second, there is a strong correlation between the average weekend day activity and the average weekday activity (Figure 4.4). It is therefore possible to identify (even screen for) the persistently sedentary child.

Conclusions and recommendations

This chapter has reviewed the metabolic implications of obesity, but can it be prevented? As far as the genetic contribution to obesity is concerned we can, as yet, do very little, although there is undoubtedly a genetic component

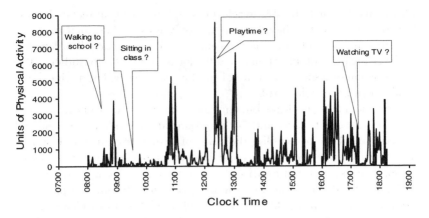

Figure 4.3 Recording of a typical day's physical activity using a CSA accelerometer.

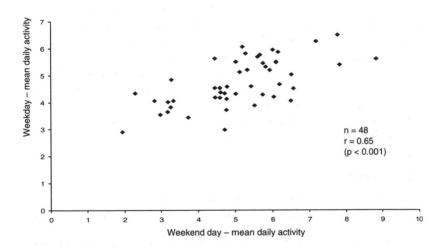

Figure 4.4 Data on physical activity from the EarlyBird Study, comparing mean weekday with mean weekend day activity.

to body shape. The fast-food culture and physical inactivity are two possible targets for intervention. However, will taking inventories of what children eat, of what physical activity they undertake, and of their body dimensions, help identify those children whose weight is associated with an unhealthy metabolic profile? All these variables are merely surrogates for the basic disturbance which is insulin resistance. A simple and non-invasive means of measuring this might be able to select out children really at metabolic risk, but for the present, a blood test is the only means. The final message, therefore, is that insulin resistance is central to obesity-related disorders. It is a direct measure of metabolic health, not a proxy like the others. The development of a simple measure of insulin resistance will be a critical step in identifying the child at risk.

These four messages leave four challenges, one to research, one to development, the third to practice and the last to education. First, resources should be made available to establish the *causes* of insulin resistance in children. This is the key to prevention. Second, biomedical science should be seeking a more precise and non-invasive means of *measuring* insulin resistance in children – for the moment, we cannot measure it with sufficient precision. Were we able to, we would have a much clearer idea as to which children were metabolically at risk of problems that will meet them later in life. Third, resources should be made available to *prevent* insulin resistance in children. This would involve teachers as well as parents and is likely to require provision of additional intra- and extra-curricular physical activity at school. The present focus on academic education may well be to the detriment of children's physical education. For the sake of their future health, this balance might need adjustment. Finally, resources should be made available to *educate* paediatricians in the risks associated with insulin resistance. Fat children are not obviously unwell and, to date, paediatricians have been largely unaware of the risks they face (Vanhala *et al.*, 1999; Ehtisham *et al.*, 2000; Drake *et al.*, 2002). Obesity is currently incubating an explosion in diabetes and other metabolic disorders. It must be tackled in childhood.

References

Bonora, E., Kiechal, S., Willeit, J., Oberhollenzer, F. *et al.* (1998) Prevalence of insulin resistance in metabolic disorders: the Bruneck Study. *Diabetes*, 47: 1643–9.

Carey, D.G., Jenkins, A.B., Campbell, L.V., Freund, J. and Chisholm, D.J. (1996) Abdominal fat and insulin resistance in normal and overweight women: direct measurements reveal a strong relationship in subjects at both low and high risk of NIDDM. *Diabetes*, 45: 633–8.

Cianfarani, S., Germani, D. and Branca, F. (1999) Low birthweight and adult insulin resistance: the 'catch-up growth' hypothesis. *Arch Dis Child Fetal Neonatal Ed*, 81, F71–3.

Drake, A.J., Smith, A., Betts, P.R., Crowne, E.C. and Shield, J.P. (2002) Type 2 diabetes in obese white children. *Arch Dis Child*, 86(3): 207–8.

Ehtisham, S., Barrett, T.G. and Shaw, N.J. (2000) Type 2 diabetes mellitus in UK children – an emerging problem. *Diabetic Med*, 17: 867–71.

Enzi, G. *et al.* (1993) Association of multiple risk factors for cardiovascular diseases and visceral obesity; a deadly quartet or sextet? In H. Ditschuneit *et al.* (eds) *Obesity in Europe.* London: Libbey, pp. 411–27.

Forsen, T., Eriksson, J., Tuomilehto, J., Reunanen, A., Osmond, C. and Barker, D. (2000) The fetal and childhood growth of persons who develop type 2 diabetes. *Ann Intern Med*, 133: 176–82.

Franks, S. (1995) Polycystic ovary syndrome. *N Engl J Med*, 333: 853–61.

Hales, C.N. and Barkerm D.J. (1992) Type 2 (non-insulin-dependent) diabetes mellitus: the thrifty phenotype hypothesis. *Diabetologia*, 35: 595–601.

Hattersley, A.T. and Tooke, J.E. (1999) The fetal insulin hypothesis: an alternative explanation of the association of low birthweight with diabetes and vascular disease. *Lancet*, 353: 1789–92

Kaaja, R., Laivuori, H., Laakso, M., Tikkanen, M.J. and Ylikorkala, O. (1999) Evidence of a state of increased insulin resistance in preeclampsia. *Metabolism*, 48: 892–6.

Lucas, A., Fewtrell, M.S. and Cole, T.J. (1999) Fetal origins of adult disease – the hypothesis revisited. *Br Med J*, 319: 245–9.

Matsuzawa, Y. (1997) Pathophysiology and molecular mechanisms of visceral fat syndrome. *Diabetes Metab Rev*, 13: 3–13.

Montague, C.T. and O'Rahilly, S. (2000) The perils of portliness: causes and consequences of visceral adiposity. *Diabetes*, 49: 883–8.

Neel, J.V. (1999) Diabetes mellitus: a 'thrifty' genotype rendered detrimental by 'progress'? *Bull World Health Organ*, 77(8): 694–703.

Prader, A. (1978) Catch-up growth. *Postgrad Med J*, 54(Suppl 1): 133–46.

Randle, P.J. (1966) Carbohydrate metabolism and lipid storage and breakdown in diabetes. *Diabetologia*, 2: 237–47.

Reaven, G.M. (1988) Banting lecture 1988. Role of insulin resistance in human disease. *Diabetes*, 37: 1595–607.

Ruderman, N., Chisholm, D., Pi-Sunyer, X. and Schneider, S. (1998) The metabolically obese, normal-weight individual revisited. *Diabetes*, 47: 699–713.

Vague, J. (1956) The degree of masculine differentiation of obesities: a factor determining predisposition to diabetes, atherosclerosis, gout and uric acid calculus disease. *Obes Res*, 4: 204–12.

Vanhala, M.J., Vanhala, P.T., Keinanen-Kiukaanniemi, S.M., Kumpusalo, E.A. and Takala, J.K. (1999) Relative weight gain and obesity as a child predict metabolic syndrome as an adult. *Int J Obes Relat Metab Disord*, 23: 656–59.

Whincup, P.H., Cook, D.G., Adshead, F., Taylor, S.J., Walker, M., Papacosta, O. and Alberti, K.G. (1997) Childhood size is more strongly related than size at birth to glucose and insulin levels in 10–11-year-old children. *Diabetologia*, 40: 319–26.

Wilkin, T.J. (1998) Endocrine feedback control in health and disease. In E.E. Bittar and N. Bittar (eds) *The Principles of Medical Biology*, Greenwich, CT: JAI Press, pp. 1–28

Zavaroni, I., Bonini, L., Gasparini, P., Barilli, A.L., Zuccarelli, A., Dall'Aglio, E., Delsignore, R. and Reaven, G.M. (1999) Hyperinsulinemia in a normal population as a predictor of non-insulin-dependent diabetes mellitus, hypertension, and coronary heart disease: the Barilla factory revisited. *Metabolism*, 48: 989–94.

Part III
Opportunities and threats

5 Social inequalities, nutrition and obesity

Suzi Leather

Introduction

As both a social scientist and Deputy Chair of the Food Standards Agency (FSA), I have a particular interest in food and health issues. The FSA is a non-ministerial Government department, headed by an independent Board, not by politicians. It was launched in April last year in response to a perceived, and indeed real, lack of public confidence in the regulation of food safety. Food issues had hitherto been dealt with by the Ministry of Agriculture, Fisheries and Food, whose responsibility it had been both to promote and regulate the food supply. The FSA now covers a wide range of issues from BSE, pesticides and dioxins to health checks in abattoirs, but nutrition is one of the most important areas of its work – a responsibility shared with the Department of Health.

It is the FSA's duty, firstly, to monitor and survey the nutrient content of food items and of the nation's diet as a whole, but its remit is also to provide *advice* on nutrition, both to consumers and to the rest of Government. In addition, we propose new legislation, represent the UK in international negotiations, formulate policy and provide advice to other government departments and commission research. The FSA is, in fact, the biggest sponsor of nutrition research, currently spending some £7 million annually in this area. There is, however, room for improvement in the way we disseminate the findings of that research and translate it into policy.

Our function, therefore, is to determine what people are *actually* eating, to recommend what people *should* eat for a balanced diet, and we also have a responsibility to *support* the public by making it easier for them to choose a balanced diet. As a medical condition, obesity is the responsibility of the Department of Health, but as a public health issue, the FSA has a major role to play in the *prevention* of obesity.

We need to be aware of the current situation and to identify any obstacles in the way of changing eating habits. We need to find out how best to educate the public, and which interventions are the most effective. The FSA is still in its infancy, but the Board is already committed to the Agency's playing a very significant role in nutrition, and an outline of our Strategic Nutrition Framework can be found on our website at www.food.gov.uk.

Social deprivation and obesity

You may already be aware of two important facts. First, there is a strong positive relationship between parental size and obesity in offspring, as there is between childhood and adult obesity. Second, both longitudinal and cross-sectional studies (Power and Parsons, 2000) show a very strong relationship between deprivation and adult obesity, in both men and women. A recent study in Plymouth (Kinra *et al.*, 2000) of some 21,000 primary school children showed a very clear association between obesity and deprivation. It also showed that the effect was particularly strong in older girls.

What are the dietary reasons for this? From the earliest years, children and parents from manual social classes are significantly disadvantaged in the quality of their diet. For a start, low-income groups are less likely to breastfeed; their poor diet continues throughout early childhood, and studies have shown clear socio-economic differences between children, even at ages 1.5 and 4.5 years old (Gregory *et al.*, 1995) (see Box 5.1). Even before these

Box 5.1   Children 1½–4½ years (1992/3)

Children from manual social class housholds *more* likely to eat:	Children from manual social class households *less* likely to eat:

• Burgers and kebabs
• Margarine
  (not polyunstaurated)
• Chips
• Table sugar
• Tea
	• Rice, wholemeal bread
	• Whole grain/high fibre
	  breakfast cereals, buns,
	  cakes and pastries
	• Butter, polyunsaturated
	  margarine, cheese,
	  fromage frais
	• Oily fish, white fish (not
	  fried)
	• Uncoated chicken
	• Raw carrots, fruit
	• Fruit juice

Source: Gregory *et al.* (1995)

children get to school and are exposed to the all-important peer pressure, they are already eating significantly more nutritionally unhealthy food than their better-off peers. In one week-long survey of older children, 20 per cent ate no fruit at all (Gregory *et al.*, 2000). The reason why the diets of poorer people are so bad is not simply a matter of income. The average household in the UK spends about £3,000 a year on food – about 16 per cent of its income after tax (Ministry of Agriculture, Fisheries and Food, 2000). The richest 20 per cent spend only 11 per cent of their net earnings on food, but the poorest 20 per cent spend considerably more – almost a third of the disposable income of poorer families goes on food. Despite this proportionately high level of expenditure on food, they are, nevertheless, not eating the quality of diet that is going to protect their long-term health.

Barriers to healthy eating

Contributory factors include not only psychosocial and educational barriers but, importantly, access to healthy food and information about food. There has been a significant increase in the number of superstores since the mid-1980s, while at the same time the number of independent neighbourhood shops has greatly declined (Box 5.2). One retailer, when asked what was the single most useful thing that Government could do to help maintain these shops said, 'Encourage local authorities to put concrete bollards around the shops so that they are not ram-raided'. The disappearance of many neigh-bourhood shops has left those without transport, the poor and the elderly, very little choice or access to fresh food. It is not easy to shop for a family in an out-of-town supermarket if you have to take one or perhaps several buses. Foot access can also be a problem in rural communities.

Another contributory factor is information. There is a huge gap between what we ought to be eating for a balanced diet and what people are actually consuming, particularly children. Research (Food Standards Agency, 2001) conducted by the FSA last year showed that less than half (only 43 per cent)

Box 5.2   Food access for low income consumers

> - People on low incomes and the elderly are more likely to shop in local shops.
> - Too many neighbourhoods have too few shops.
> - Local shops are less likely to stock fresh fruit and vegetables, and cannot compete with supermarket prices.
> - Growth of out-of-town retailing combined with poor, inadequate transport links in deprived areas has exacerbated the problem.

the population are *aware* of the 'eat five portions of fruit or vegetables a day' message and, of those, only 26 per cent thought they had actually done so the day before. One reason why these guidelines are still largely ignored is because health is boring, but there are also some very effective counter-messages to healthy eating. The advertising budget for the kinds of foods that dominate children's diets is enormous and raises questions as to how this contributes to the current and future obesity problem we are witnessing. A huge amount of money (around £70m) is spent on promoting foods that are high in fat, salt and sugar while, by contrast, the Health Development Agency has a total budget of only £750,000. It is hardly surprising, therefore, that even those in the top income bracket in the UK do not consume the WHO recommended amount of fruit and vegetables (World Health Organization, 1990). It is of particular concern that those in the lower groups eat barely half the amount of fruit and vegetables recommended to protect health (Figure 5.1). The so-called 'nutrition gap' in society is growing wider, precisely for the foods people need to be eating more of in order to substitute for foods they should be eating less of. The FSA aims not only to achieve a long-term improvement in the nutrition of the UK population as a whole, but also to see a reduction in inequalities by enabling and encouraging disadvantaged people to improve their diets.

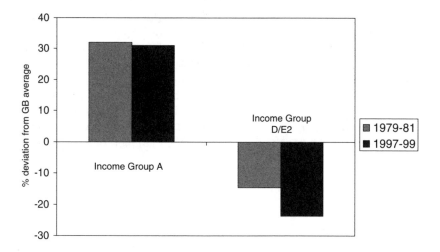

Figure 5.1 Trends in consumption of fresh fruit by income group (A versus D/E2) of GB average, 1979–81 and 1997–9[a] (Source: MAFF National Food Survey, 2000).

Note: a = based on head of household income.

Strategies to reduce the 'nutrition gap'

Strategies need firstly to be evidence-based, and this requires some robust baseline data on the nutritional status of low-income groups. There has not been a specific low-income survey on diets since the 1930s (Boyd Orr, 1937), but the FSA is now commissioning such a piece of research, to be published in 2005. It will include, not only dietary assessment and blood and urine samples, but also some aspects of social exclusion that go beyond simply low income. The proposed research will explore some of the reasons why people find it difficult, psychologically as well as practically, to make the recommended dietary changes, and even why some may feel that healthy eating messages do not apply to them.

Some important intervention work under the Agency's food acceptability and choice research programme, such as the 'Cook Well' initiative, has begun in terms of teaching culinary skills. If we are trying to move away from high-fat, high-sugar and high-salt processed foods, it is important that we retain the ability to cook from fresh. It is essential that this skill is not lost, and we are currently running a project in Scotland to improve cooking skills and observe the impact on nutritional status. We are also conducting a study in Newcastle, on the subject of so-called 'food deserts', much spoken about but until now an under-researched area. As far as the prevention of obesity in childhood is concerned, there are some family and school interventions currently under way in Oxford.

We believe that food education is extremely important and we have been very supportive of the British Nutrition Foundation's efforts to further develop material for schools. It would help to put practical cooking skills back into the national curriculum. Increasingly, however, people are choosing to eat outside the home, where they have little or no control over what goes into their food. The FSA is therefore supporting a 'Catering for Health' initiative (Food Standards Agency/Department of Health, 2001), which is training those responsible for public and private sector catering to have some understanding of nutrition and the need for more healthy menus (Box 5.3).

Box 5.3 Catering for health

- Guidelines developed by the British Nutrition Foundation, with FSA and DoH support.
- Information and practical ideas for chef lecturers and caterers about how healthier catering practices can be implemented in all aspects of catering, in a wide range of working environments.

Importantly, we are trying to get nutrition built into the syllabus for students of catering as well as medicine and other allied professions.

There is evidence that we need to target children and young people in care. Their access to adequate health care, and health care information, is often very poor, and many of them arrive in care having experienced poor nutrition as well as considerable deprivation. Even in care they are often no better off nutritionally. We are therefore developing an initiative with Department of Health and British Nutrition Foundation, through the Caroline Walker Trust, to improve the diets of such children (Box 5.4). We hope soon to put a document into every residential home in the country in order to target this particularly vulnerable group.

One of the first goals of the FSA was to improve nutritional labelling in the UK. In comparison to the range of products carrying nutrition labelling in the US, food labelling in Europe is woefully inadequate. Unfortunately, improvement will not happen overnight because, as in many other areas of food legislation, the direction comes from Brussels. Initially, any changes are likely to be made on a voluntary basis; in the long-term, a change in the law will probably be required.

The issue of food promotion to children is important. One only has to watch television on a Saturday morning to see this – the amount of money spent on advertisements for high-fat, high-salt and high-sugar foods is huge. Moreover, the messages run absolutely counter to all the healthy eating advice. More than 70 per cent of television advertisements aimed at children are for such foods, so children are a very important target group for these advertisers. Of course, there is always a balance to be struck between the needs of the manufacturing industries and the health of the nation. Nevertheless, faced with the rise in obesity and the diet-related health problems

Box 5.4   Eating well for children and young people in care

Partly funded by the FSA, the Caroline Walker Trust has produced guidelines for all those involved in providing care for this particularly vulnerable group.

- Provides advice for developing suitable, nutritionally balanced menus.
- Gives background to the relationship between nutrition, physical activity and health.
- Practical advice to help develop the food skills needed by young people for life after care.

that we now have, we have to consider how best to serve the interests of our children's health.

One role of the FSA is to set up an evidence base for measures that work. Very little work, to date, has gone into evaluating nutritional interventions, for example. There is a particular need to have national co-ordination because there is currently a plethora of health improvement schemes: National Service Frameworks, Sure Start, Health Action Zones, and so on. In order to run a successful health improvement programme, one has to know what to include. It clearly must include nutrition and must certainly target communities with the worst diets. Community food projects are important and should be actively supported and encouraged by health professionals. We need new food and nutrition posts in the community and in the Health Action Zones, where to date the professional infrastructure has been quite inadequate.

Finally, in both primary and secondary care, there is an urgent need for better service provision. While the focus must always remain on prevention, the facts are that we now have an estimated 4.2 million obese women and 3.2 million obese men in the UK, but only twelve obesity clinics (Auditor General, 2001) – an astonishing gap between demand and supply. It is one of the duties of the FSA to develop national guidance as to where we go from here.

References

Auditor General (2001) *Tackling Obesity in England. Report by the Comptroller and Auditor General.* HC 220 Session 2000–2001, 15 February 2001.

Boyd Orr, J. (1937) *Food, Health and Income. Report on Survey of Adequacy of Diet in Relation to Income,* 2nd edn. London: Macmillan.

Food Standards Agency (2001) *Consumer Attitudes to Food Standards Final Report January 2001.* Surveyed over 3,100 people in the UK between October and December 2000. A copy of the report is available on the Agency's Website: http://www. foodstandards.gov.uk/pdf files/consumer.pdf.

Food Standards Agency/Department of Health (2001) *Catering for Health. A Guide for Teaching Healthier Catering Practices.* London: Food Standards Agency and Department of Health.

Gregory, J., Collins, D.L., Davies, P.S.W., Hughes, J.M. and Clarke, P.C. (1995) *National Diet and Nutrition Survey; Children Aged 1½–4½ Years, Volume 1: Report of the Diet and Nutrition Survey.*

Gregory, J., Lowe, S., Bates, C.J., Prentice, A., Jackson, L.V., Smithers, G., Wenlock, R. and Farron, M. (2000) *National Diet and Nutrition Survey: Young People Aged 4 to 18 Years, Volume 1: Report of the Diet and Nutrition Survey.*

Kinra, S., Nelder, R.P. and Lewendon, G.J. (2000) Deprivation and childhood obesity: a cross sectional study of 20,973 children in Plymouth, United Kingdom. *J Epidemiol Community Health,* 54(6): 456–60.

Ministry of Agriculture, Fisheries and Foods (2000) *National Food Survey 2000*. Annual Report on Food Expenditure, Consumption and Nutrient Intakes. London: The Stationery Office.

Power, C. and Parsons, T. (2000) Nutritional and other influences in childhood as predictors of adult obesity. *Proc Nutr Soc*, 59(2): 267–72.

World Health Organization (1990) *Diet, Nutrition and the Prevention of Diseases*. WHO Technical Report Series 1990 (797). Geneva: World Health Organization.

6   Self-image and the stigma of obesity

Andrew J. Hill

Weight is a major determinant of self-perception and self-esteem, and there is good evidence that both adults and children are stigmatized and mistreated if they are overweight. Although attitudes towards obesity are shaped by age, gender and cultural background, negative attitudes are pervasive. These anti-fat attitudes lead to assumptions about the character and psychological state of obese people and are linked, in turn, to prevailing Western attitudes about responsibility and blame. Our portrayal of obesity, understanding of its causes and approaches to treatment need to acknowledge properly the influence of an obesogenic environment, and not be based on a misconceived notion of will power.

The social meaning of obesity

Cross-culturally, the meaning of obesity is determined by values within a society about what constitutes a normal body shape, how beauty is recognized and whether body weight has any implications for health. Health is a fairly new obesity-related issue as Western medicine has only recently begun to recognize the associations between obesity and impaired physical health. Past attributions of health to fat infants, often voiced by grandparents, have been replaced by concerns about persistent future obesity.

Perceptions of body size are also loosely related to the affluence of a particular culture. In poor countries, plumpness, though rarely frank obesity, is favoured and is regarded as a sign of wealth or status. Richer nations, on the other hand, prize thinness. The resultant observation is that societies favour the body shape that is most difficult to attain. Moreover, the importance of body shape and appearance generally applies more to women than to men. It is for these reasons that women in Western societies report such high levels of body shape and weight concern.

Obesity and stereotyping

Children are very frank as far as their perception of obesity is concerned. Numerous studies have shown children to associate fatness with low intelligence, laziness, social isolation and unattractiveness. More recent research has extended this characterization and shows that even pre-adolescents have incorporated the message of poor health, fitness and failure to eat healthily in their attributions of overweight (Hill and Silver, 1995). Adults share this stereotyping, seeing obese people as undisciplined, inactive, unappealing and with emotional or psychological problems. Only one positive quality is part of the obesity stereotype: obese people are seen as more humorous, funny and warm. But even this can be demeaning to seriously obese individuals when, in reality, this may be the last thing they feel like.

Very little research has looked at the characteristics of people who are most likely to stereotype. What exists suggests that negative stereotyping is more likely in people who are leaner, younger, female, of higher socio-economic background and who are non-health professionals (Robinson *et al.*, 1993). These, however, are just moderating factors. There is evidence that some doctors, nurses, dietitians and psychologists also hold negative stereotyped views of obesity (Harvey and Hill, 2001). This is not to blame the medical profession for these particular attitudes. The evidence simply reflects the case that medical training does not give immunity to the values and views that are prevalent in society. Anti-fat attitudes are widely held and they are overt (Crandall, 1994). Unlike racism, which tends to be suppressed in public, it is quite acceptable to be 'weightist', to show pictures of female celebrities and comment on their size and shape, unattractiveness and personality flaws.

Obesity, anxiety and depression

The presence of anxiety and/or depression in obese clinical groups has been repeatedly researched. The older research literature is inconclusive regarding the relationship between obesity and anxiety/depression. Prevalence estimates of emotional disturbance have varied widely, in part due to the large differences between studies.

One of the common problems is that of sample size. Very few studies have managed to gather data from a sufficiently large sample of obese people. The Swedish Obese Subjects (SOS) intervention study is an exception, and a relatively recent one at that. This evaluation of gastric surgical treatment for obesity has included psychological measures alongside physical and medical outcomes. The baseline evaluation of the first 1,700 patients showed much higher levels of emotional disorders than in healthy lean people

(Sullivan *et al.*, 1993). Obese men (mean body mass index (BMI) = 34 kg/m²) and women (38 kg/m²) both scored higher than lean controls on a self-report measure of anxiety and depression. The obese were over four times more likely to have clinical anxiety and seven times more likely to be clinically depressed.

Two notes of caution are warranted. First, clinical samples consistently score higher than community samples in terms of psychological and psychiatric problems. This applies across a range of health issues, not just overweight and obesity. We attempted to address this by recruiting a community sample from the readership of a specialist magazine published for larger women (Hill and Williams, 1998). Of the 70 respondents with a BMI above 40, over 40 per cent reported past episodes of anxiety and nearly 50 per cent past depression. However, this was not reliably higher than the levels seen in women with lesser grades of obesity or who were simply overweight. It should also be recognized that population levels of depression are high. In the UK 10 per cent of adults are depressed in any week, and 55 per cent at some time in their lives (Davies and Craig, 1998).

Second, prevalence estimates vary according to the method of assessment. Self-reports and questionnaire measures tend to overestimate the presence of clinical anxiety and depression. Probably the best evidence so far comes from an analysis of the 1992 National Longitudinal Alcohol Epidemiologic Survey, which involved a structured diagnostic interview of over 40,000 US adults (Carpenter *et al.*, 2000). As Table 6.1 shows, obesity was associated with an *increased* risk of depression among women but a *decreased* risk of depression in men. Quantifying this, for women being obese was associated with a 37 per cent increase in the odds of being diagnosed with major depression, while obese men were 37 per cent less likely to be so diagnosed. There was a similar association between obesity, gender and suicide attempts

Table 6.1 Adjusted odds ratios for the association of weight status and psychiatric outcome in women and men

| | Obese vs average weight | |
	Women	Men
Major depression OR (95% CI)	1.37 (1.09, 1.73)	0.63 (0.60, 0.67)
Suicide ideation OR (95% CI)	1.20 (0.96, 1.50)	1.02 (0.98, 1.06)
Suicide attempts OR (95% CI)	1.23 (0.74, 2.03)	0.63 (0.48, 0.83)

Source: Carpenter *et al.* (2000)

– obese women were at increased risk, obese men at decreased risk. Furthermore, although the association between female obesity and depression was rather modest in epidemiological terms, the authors had controlled for depression co-occurring with physical illness or bereavement. When they included the latter, the association between obesity and past-year depression further strengthened.

The present evidence suggests therefore that anxiety and depression are over-represented in obese people seeking clinical assistance relative to community samples. Obese women may be more at risk of anxiety and depression than obese men.

Obesity and emotional well-being

Further studies of large representative samples using established measures of well-being have helped separate physical functioning from psychological health, while also showing their interdependence. In one ongoing project, Brown and colleagues have examined the relationship between BMI, health and well-being from data collected as part of the Australian Longitudinal Study on Women's Health. They, like others, have used the SF-36, a questionnaire that assesses eight dimensions of subjective health status and two summary physical and mental health components.

Analysis of the 14,000 women in the younger age group (18–23 years) showed both overweight and obese women to score significantly lower in physical functioning, vitality and general health (Brown *et al.*, 2000). There were no differences in any of the main psychological health measures. The pattern for middle age women (45–49 years) was different (Brown *et al.*, 1998). For a start, there were substantially more overweight and obese women in this cohort. Moreover, these older obese women scored significantly lower than those of average weight on all of the physical and psychological health scales, and the greatest deficits were seen in those who were the heaviest.

Another study has used the SF-36 to look at UK adults (Doll *et al.*, 2000). Again, the obese scored lower than their normal-weight counterparts on every scale. The most severely obese (BMI>40) scored the lowest of all groups. Interestingly, for all of the psychological health scales the moderately obese (BMI 30–40) were statistically similar to the under-weight (BMI<18.5), whereas the overweight were similar to normal weight individuals. The data were not analysed to compare men and women, or young and old. The authors, however, did examine the co-occurrence of chronic illness. People with obesity plus other chronic health conditions (around half of the obese) reported particularly poor physical and psychological health. Since this was most apparent in those with three or more chronic conditions it identifies an especially vulnerable group. It is also notable that, among groups of people with similar levels of chronic illness, the additional presence of obesity was associated with a significant deterioration in physical but not emotional well-being (Figure 6.1). This means that past assessments of psychological well-being may have been confounded by physical health problems. It also shows that obese individuals with multiple co-occurring chronic illnesses are most at risk of psychological distress.

Cause or consequence?

Virtually all research evidence in this area derives from cross-sectional studies, making conclusions about causality very difficult. Does being obese make people depressed, or does being depressed lead to weight gain and obesity? The answer is that the relationship is probably circular. The most favoured mechanisms for the association include both the stigma associated with obesity in Western culture and the greater tendency for the obese to eat in response to negative emotions. However, the risk to psychological health when obesity co-occurs with chronic illness suggests a pathway to problems that is common to many disabilities. This takes into account the social repercussions of having a highly visible, stigmatized condition and the resultant effect on self-esteem.

Self-esteem

The relationship between obesity and self-esteem is again not straightforward. In adults, obesity is associated with a modest reduction in self-esteem,

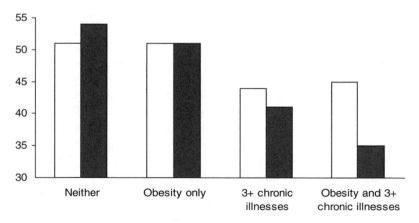

Figure 6.1 Mean mental health (white columns) and physical health (shaded columns) component scores from the SF-36 in adults with and without obesity and chronic illnesses (Source: Doll *et al.*, 2000).

sometimes limited only to those with morbid obesity (Miller and Downey, 1999). In pre-adolescent children, obesity has little or no impact on global self-esteem (French *et al.*, 1995). In older age groups, self-perceived overweight is more closely associated with reduced self-esteem than is actual overweight. Similarly, this relationship is stronger in women than in men.

Body esteem, or satisfaction with appearance, is the domain of self-worth most affected by obesity. This is especially true for obese adolescent and young women whose sense of identity is dependent on appearance and some of whom show very high levels of body dissatisfaction. Again, body dissatisfaction may be more strongly associated with perceived overweight and depression than with actual weight. Therapy aimed at improving body image in obese women has shown some success in relieving negative psychological symptoms but has little impact on body weight (Rosen *et al.*, 1995).

Social consequences

Conceptualizations of self-esteem argue that it is a socially derived state, being the product of perceived competence in areas deemed personally (and culturally) important, together with the approval of significant others in one's life. Social rejection is faced by many obese people, whether the experience is actual or anticipated. The SOS surgical intervention study included questions on social activities and interactions (Sullivan *et al.*, 1993). A high proportion of patients reported being 'mostly' or 'definitely bothered' about social activities especially if the respondent was female and if they were in public. So, for example, being bothered about (and so generally avoiding) going out to a restaurant was reported by nearly two-thirds of women, holidaying away from home by over a half, and buying clothes or public bathing by nearly 90 per cent. In our own study of magazine readers, low self-esteem and poor peer relationships were both predictors of poor mental health (Hill and Williams, 1998). In contrast, degree of obesity, weight history and eating behaviour (dieting or binge eating) were not.

Box 6.1 summarizes the most frequently encountered stigmatizing situations reported by a sample of obese Americans (Myers and Rosen, 1999). Although such situations were encountered on average less than once per year, they describe the variety of interpersonal and environmental challenges faced. That these include comments from doctors, family, children and strangers should not come as a surprise given the previous commentary. Overall, some 40 per cent of US obese adults report having experienced weight-related mistreatment, over half of them from their spouse and two-thirds from strangers (Falkner *et al.*, 1999). Being fat makes a person public property, permitting anyone to pass judgement on the cause of their obesity and the necessary remedy.

Box 6.1

---

1 Comments from children:
  'As an adult, having a child make fun of you'.
  'A child coming up to you and saying someting like "You're fat!".'

2 Others making negative assumptions about you:
  'Other people having low expectations of you because of your weight'.
  'Having people assume you have emotional problems because you are overweight'.

3 Physical barriers:
  'Not being able to fit into seats at restaurants, theatres and other public places'.
  'Not being able to find clothes that fit'.

4 Being stared at:
  'Being stared at in public'.
  'Groups of people pointing and laughing at you in public'.

5 Inappropriate comments from doctors:
  'Having a doctor make cruel remarks, ridicule you, or call you names'.
  'A doctor blaming unrelated physical problems on your weight'.

6 Nasty comments from family:
  'A spouse/partner calling you names because of your weight'.
  'A parent or other relative nagging you to lose weight'.

7 Nasty comments from other:
  'Having strangers suggest diets to you'.
  'Being offered fashion advice from strangers'.

8 Being avoided, excluded, ignored:
  'Being unable to get a date because of your size'.
  'Being singled out as a child by a teacher, school nurse, etc., because of your size'.

Source: Meyers and Rosen (1999)

Children are part of this persecutory milieu. They stigmatize on the basis of appearance and in turn are stigmatized for overweight. So-called 'fat teasing' has been examined in young adolescent children in the UK (Hill and Murphy, 2000). Twelve per cent of girls and 16 per cent of boys reported being teased or bullied for their overweight. Although these victimized children were heavier than their non-victimized peers, fewer than half were overweight or obese. Fat teasing was associated with low body-shape satisfaction and low self-esteem. Girls victimized for overweight were the most likely to be dissatisfied with their physical appearance, and nearly 50 per cent had already tried dieting to lose weight. The levels of fat teasing at primary school age appear to be even higher at nearly one in five children (Waterston and Hill, 2002). In addition, being teased about being fat is viewed as one of the worst things to be teased for at this age.

Such victimization is not a benign experience. Myers and Rosen (1999) found that stigmatization frequency was in negative correlation with measures of mental health, body dissatisfaction and self-esteem. These associations were still present when BMI was included as a covariate. In other words, it was the frequency of these events that was important.

Obesity and discrimination

Stereotyping leads to prejudice and ultimately to discrimination. Research into discrimination has frequently used simulated employment decisions. In one such study, overweight candidates were less likely to be hired even though they were perceived equally competent on job-related tests as non-obese candidates (Larkin and Pines, 1979). In another, public health administrators were sent a letter asking for information about the prospects of establishing a career in the health profession. The overweight applicant received fewer responses than the normal-weight applicant. Even when they received a reply, they were seen as less likely to get into a graduate programme and get a good job after training (Benson et al., 1980). In a study controlling for facial attractiveness, college students were less likely to hire an overweight applicant in a position involving sales, and therefore interaction with the public, but equally likely to hire if it was a business position (Rothblum et al., 1988). Finally, adults with employment experience were asked to make recruitment decisions and personal judgements on the basis of job descriptions, resumés and short videotaped interviews (Klesges et al., 1990). Both obese and diabetic applicants were less likely to be hired, but for different perceived reasons. The obese applicant, for example, was viewed as having poor work habits and more likely to have emotional and interpersonal problems.

Although methodological criticisms have been levelled at some of these studies, their outcome is in accord with the personal experience of some obese individuals in the job sector. Reduced employment prospects may be an example of the real-life penalties of obesity, along with discrimination in the areas of education and health care (Puhl and Brownell, 2001). This is supported by analyses of large survey databases. Overweight and obese young adult women in the US and UK earn significantly less than non-overweight women or those with other chronic health problems (Gortmaker *et al.*, 1993; Sargent and Blanchflower, 1994). This is not the case for men. Additionally, US adolescent women with a BMI above the 95th percentile were found seven years later to have completed fewer years of school, they were less likely to be married, and they had higher rates of household poverty, independent of their teenage socio-economic status. Similarly categorized men were only less likely to be married.

Focusing specifically on women's employment, Cawley (2000) has looked again at the National Longitudinal Survey of Youth, a sample of nearly 13,000 young people designed to represent the entire population of American youth in 1979 (the sample reported on by Gortmaker *et al.* in 1993). Looking at hourly wages, employment and sector of occupation, Cawley found that women who were heavier earned less. A difference of two standard deviations from the mean sample weight was associated with a reduction in wages of seven per cent. In absolute value, this was equivalent to one year of education, two years of job tenure or three years of work experience. This applied to white women but not to Hispanic or black women. The impact of overweight on wages was not seen either in likelihood of employment or in sector of occupation. For white US women, at least, obesity costs.

Responsibility and blame

Attitudes to obesity in the Western world are linked, inextricably, to the notion that somehow the individual is to blame for his or her obesity. Crandall (1994) argues that this ideology of blame is a function of two components. First, there is a cultural preference for thinness, and second, it is believed that weight is under voluntary control. The former is undeniably true. The latter is less certain, judging by the experience of most people who try to lose weight. It is hard to believe that the prevalence of obesity has tripled in the past 20 years because people have deliberately decided to gain weight. Rather, there has been a steady increase in the sales of diet products running concurrently with the increase in the prevalence of obesity. Yet the diet sector appears to have done little to put a brake on the epidemic.

Governmentally-set targets to reduce obesity, such as the UK's Health of the Nation 1992 White Paper, have fostered the notion that individual choice is the key to implementing behavioural change. People are urged to become more physically active and to eat less. Obesity, it is implied, is a modifiable risk factor. However, making obesity a lifestyle disorder has helped hardly anybody. Instead, it has inflamed anti-fat attitudes and the prejudice directed at the obese. The prevailing Western ideology, epitomized by the US but shared by other Western nations, is that each person is responsible for what they get in life. This emphasis on individual responsibility and self-determination enables any US citizen to aspire to become president. It is the basis of will power. It also permits the belief that people get what they deserve and deserve what they get. Thus, poor people are held responsible for their own poverty, drug users for their addiction, and fat people for their obesity (Crandall and Schiffhauer, 1998). Unsurprisingly, the more people endorse absence of will power as a cause of obesity, the greater their anti-fat attitudes and prejudice (Crandall, 1994).

Conclusions

For many people, their obesity is not under their volitional control, biologically or psychologically. Victim-blaming fosters stigmatization and prejudice, and the more people are stigmatized, the lower their self-esteem. Respect from others is what gives us our sense of self-worth and self-esteem. One of the prerequisites to behavioural change is the confidence that it can be done, and confidence can only come from self-esteem. With confidence comes self-efficacy, but without it, no amount of dietary advice will have any effect.

To make change happen requires a shift away from the traditional view that obesity is a personal disorder that requires treatment. It is an international disorder, considered by some a pandemic. The task of anyone looking to promote a more healthy weight is to understand how behaviour is constrained by its environment. Obesity is not an abnormal response to a normal environment; it is a normal response to an abnormal environment (Egger and Swinburn, 1997). Over the last 20–30 years the environmental changes that influence food intake and physical activity have been multiple, unseen and concerted in a direction that fosters weight gain. The challenge for those working to treat and prevent obesity will be to alter this obesogenic environment and enable lifestyle choice. At a personal level we should be looking to empower, not blame, to bolster confidence and self-esteem, not vilify for lack of will power.

References

Benson, P.L., Severs, D., Tatgenhorst, J. and Loddengaard, N. (1980) The social costs of obesity: a non-reactive field study. *Soc Behav Pers*, 8: 91–6.

Brown, W.J., Dobson, A.J. and Mishra, G. (1998) What is a healthy weight for middle-aged women? *Int J Obesity*, 22: 520–8.

Brown, W.J., Mishra, G., Kenardy, J. and Dobson, A. (2000) Relationships between body mass index and well-being in young Australian women. *Int J Obesity*, 24: 1360–8.

Carpenter, K.M., Hasin, D.S., Allison, D.B. and Faith, M.S. (2000) Relationship between obesity and DSM-IV major depressive disorder, suicide ideation, and suicide attempts: Results from a general population study. *Am J Pub Health*, 90: 251–7.

Cawley, J. (2000) *Body Weight and Women's Labour Market Outcomes*. National Bureau of Economic Research Working Paper 7841. Cambridge, MA: National Bureau of Economic Research (Available online: http://www.nber.org/papers/w7841).

Crandall, C.S. (1994) Prejudice against fat people: ideology and self-interest. *J Pers Soc Psychol*, 66: 882–94.

Crandall, C.S. and Schiffhauer, K.L. (1998) Anti-fat prejudice: beliefs, values, and American culture. *Obesity Res*, 6: 458–60.

Davies, T. and Craig, T.K.J. (eds) (1998) *ABC of Mental Health*. London: BMJ Books.

Doll, H.A., Petersen, S.E.K. and Stewart-Brown, S.L. (2000) Obesity and physical and emotional well-being: associations between body mass index, chronic illness, and the physical and mental components of the SF-36 questionnaire. *Obesity Res*, 8: 160–70.

Egger, G. and Swinburn, B. (1997) An 'ecological' approach to the obesity pandemic. *Br Med J*, 315: 477–80.

Falkner, N.H., French, S.A., Jeffery, R.W., Neumark-Sztainer, D., Sherwood, N.E. and Morton, N. (1999) Mistreatment due to weight: prevalence and sources of perceived mistreatment in women and men. *Obesity Res*, 7: 572–6.

French, S.A., Story, M. and Perry, C.L. (1995) Self-esteem and obesity in children and adolescents: a literature review. *Obesity Res*, 3: 479–90.

Gortmaker, S.L., Must, A., Perrin, J.M., Sobol, A.M. and Dietz, W.H. (1993) Social and economic consequences of overweight in adolescence and young adulthood. *N Engl J Med*, 329: 1008–12.

Harvey, E.L. and Hill, A.J. (2001) Health professionals' views of overweight people and smokers. *Int J Obes*, 25: 1253–61.

Hill, A.J. and Murphy, J.A. (2000) The psycho-social consequences of fat-teasing in young adolescent children. *Int J Obes*, 24(Suppl. 1): 161.

Hill, A.J. and Silver, E. (1995) Fat, friendless and unhealthy: 9-year-old children's perception of body shape stereotypes. *Int J Obes*, 19: 423–30.

Hill, A.J. and Waterston, C.L. (2002) Fat-teasing in pre-adolescent children: the bullied and the bullies. *Int J Obes*, 26(Suppl. 1): 20.

Hill, A.J. and Williams, J. (1998) Psychological health in a non-clinical sample of obese women. *Int J Obes*, 22: 578–83.

Klesges, R.C., Klem, M.L., Hanson, C.L., Eck, L.H., Ernst, J., O'Laughlin, D., Garrott, A. and Rife, R. (1990) The effects of applicant's health status and qualifications on simulated hiring decisions. *Int J Obes*, 14: 527–35.

Larkin, J.C. and Pines, H.A. (1979) No fat persons need apply: experimental studies of the overweight stereotype and hiring preference. *Sociol Work Occup*, 6: 312–27.

Miller, C.T. and Downey, K.T. (1999) A meta-analysis of heavyweight and self-esteem. *Pers Soc Psychol Rev*, 3: 68–84.

Myers, A. and Rosen, J.C. (1999) Obesity stigmatization and coping: Relation to mental health symptoms, body image, and self-esteem. *Int J Obes*, 23: 221–30.

Puhl, R. and Brownell, K.D. (2001) Bias, discrimination and obesity. *Obes Res*, 9: 788–805.

Robinson, B.E., Bacon, J.G. and O'Reilly, J. (1993) Fat phobia: measuring, understanding, and changing anti-fat attitudes. *Int J Eating Disord*, 14: 467–80.

Rosen, J.C., Orosan, P. and Reiter, J. (1995) Cognitive behaviour therapy for negative body image in obese women. *Behav Therapy*, 26: 25–42.

Rothblum, E.D., Miller, C.T. and Garbutt, B. (1988) Stereotypes of obese job applicants. *Int J Eat Disord*, 7: 277–83.

Sargent, J.D. and Blanchflower, D.G. (1994) Obesity and stature in adolescence and earnings in young adulthood. Analysis of a British birth cohort. *Arch Ped Adoles Med*, 148: 681–7.

Sullivan, M., Karlsson, J., Sjöström, L. *et al.* (1993) Swedish obese subjects (SOS) – an intervention study of obesity. Baseline evaluation of health and psychosocial functioning in the first 1743 subjects examined. *Int J Obes*, 17: 503–12.

7 The view from primary care

Ian Campbell

As a general practitioner, I shall be considering in this paper how obesity relates to primary care. I will also touch on why I became enthusiastic about managing it, and why I think that others in primary care should be enthusiastic too. I want also to talk about my feelings of pride and my feelings about prejudice. I am proud about the way primary care deals with so many problems in the face of limited resources and increasing workload, but I also want to talk about the prejudice seen in primary care towards the obese, the same prejudice that one finds throughout society towards the obese. I have become convinced, over recent years, that obesity is a major threat to the health of our nation. Rather than talk about the global epidemic, however, I want to show you what it means for the individual patient.

Alison's story

I want to tell you about Alison. She is a normal 31-year-old lady, married, with two children. She works in a factory making swimming costumes and two years ago her weight was 122 kg. Her body mass index (BMI) was 44. Alison came to see me because she suffered greatly from a lack of self-esteem and was depressed. Although she had had various treatments for her so-called 'postnatal depression', she could not find a way out of her current despair. We suspected that the underlying problem was, perhaps, her obesity and put her on a weight management programme, involving dietary, exercise and behavioural changes. In February 1999 she weighed 122 kg. By June 2000 she was down to 68.5 kg, and by the following April, she weighed 77.4 kg. She is exceptional, but her case proves the point that it is possible to help people lose weight in general practice. Not only did her weight change, but so too did her outlook on life. She began to take an interest in what she was wearing and was recently caught at a children's party, playing on the bouncy castle. She is just full of life and very happy with herself. Her husband too is proud of what she has achieved for herself. In Alison's words 'I've got my life back'. That is what you can do for people in primary care.

The pattern of Alison's weight loss shows that it dipped rapidly over the first 12 months, settled and then climbed slightly. Because she had learned how to control her weight, however, she has been able to maintain the weight loss and not regain it. Some 2 years later, she is continuing to exercise three times a week. That is the story of just one patient and there is so much more to do. One in every two adults, men and women, is overweight. The problem is all around us and is inescapable.

The burden of obesity in primary care

What is the burden of obesity in primary care? As Figure 7.1 shows, the prevalence of overweight and obesity in the UK has risen dramatically over the last two decades. Aside from the increased workload, we can also identify a 30 per cent increase in prescription rates. Now, over any 5-year period, 95 per cent of my patients will come through the surgery door, for a variety or reasons. This provides a perfect opportunity to identify and tackle this problem.

If people want to be overweight and are happy with their appearance, why should the general practitioner be bothered? We *should* be bothered, not about the cosmetic effects of obesity, but about its medical effects. Type 2 diabetes is a major and growing problem. Figures produced by the National Audit Office from European and North American data show that obese women, for example, have a nearly 13 per cent increased risk of type 2 diabetes (Table 7.1.) (Chan *et al.*, 1994). For men it is only a little less. Once BMI rises above 30, the rate increases rapidly. The risk of developing diabetes

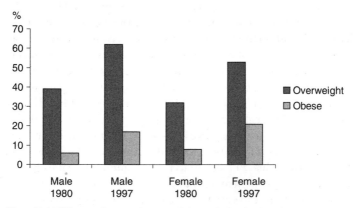

Figure 7.1 UK prevalence of overweight and obesity in adults.

Table 7.1 Increased risk for obese developing disease

Disease	Relative risk	
	Women	Men
Type 2 diabetes	12.7	5.2
Hypertension	4.2	2.6
Myocardial infarct	3.2	1.5
Cancer of the colon	2.7	3.0
Angina	1.8	1.8
Gall bladder disease	1.8	1.8
Ovarian cancer	1.7	–
Osteoarthritis	1.4	1.9
Stroke	1.3	1.3

Source: Chan *et al.* (1994)

with a BMI of 24.9 – still within 'normal' weight range – is double that of a person whose BMI is 23. The so-called 'metabolic syndrome', hyperglycaemia, hypertension, hyperlipidaemia, cardiovascular disease, these are all part of an average day's work for a general practitioner, yet obesity is the underlying factor. Angina, gall bladder disease, ovarian and colonic cancer, osteoarthritis, respiratory disease and stroke – all are related to obesity (Pi-Sunyer, 1993). Obesity is now the biggest preventable cause of cancer in non-smoking adults (Adami *et al.*, 2001). It is probably the major risk factor for hypertension and cardiovascular disease. These are the effects of obesity and this is what motivates me as a general practitioner, whether I recognize obesity as an underlying cause of it or not. It is of concern that some doctors and some nurses still dispute the fact that obesity is a medical problem. Perhaps if they recognized the problem, they would feel obliged to tackle it.

The total costs of obesity are incalculable, whether direct or indirect. A conservative estimate for the UK in 1998 was some £500 million, and similar or even higher figures are reported elsewhere (National Audit Office, 2001). Indirect costs are harder to measure but would include disability, earlier pensionable retirement and poorer education. In the UK, in 1998, 18 million sick days – that is 40,000 years of working life – were lost on account of obesity-related factors (National Audit Office, 2001). On average, those with obesity-related disease die nine years early. These are costs we can attempt to measure. There are others that we cannot measure – the shame, the loss of self-esteem, the social isolation, the loss of employment and travel opportunities. A person with a BMI of 40 cannot physically fit into a regular aeroplane seat, yet is unlikely to be able to afford a first-class seat. If they are not unemployed, they are likely to be in a relatively low paid job. Lest we forget, these are intangible, but very real costs.

In my practice, and it is of average size, I have 40 type 2 diabetics. Ninety per cent of them are overweight, two-thirds are obese. The standard treatment is to give tablets to control their blood sugar, but treating them with tablets is just a surrogate for losing weight. To make matters worse, most of these tablets will increase their weight.

What priority obesity?

If we were able to help people lose weight, would it make a difference? There is evidence to suggest that a 10 per cent weight loss can lead to a 30 per cent fall in diabetes-related deaths and a 40 per cent fall in other obesity related deaths (Table 7.2) (Goldstein, 1992). It can lower blood pressure by some 10 mmHg (systolic)/20 mmHg (diastolic), fasting glucose by *50 per cent*, total cholesterol by 10 per cent, and it can increase high-density lipoprotein cholesterol by 8 per cent (Goldstein, 1992). All this can be achieved by a mere 10 per cent weight loss which is achievable and sustainable.

When I asked why obesity has been largely ignored in the National Service Framework for Coronary Heart Disease, a senior manager from the Department of Health said that it was due to a 'managerial oversight'. Obesity is given the lowest priority. By April 2001, all NHS groups were supposed to have developed an obesity management strategy, but it did not happen. By April 2002, we were supposed to have quantifiable data as to what steps have been taken and what has been achieved.

NICE, the National Institute of Clinical Excellence, does now recognize obesity as a problem, and it even recognizes that doctors and nurses need more training. Exceptionally, it recognizes that the cost of treating obesity must go up. This has led to increased expectation from patients and health authorities, and primary care trusts are starting to develop their strategies,

Table 7.2 Benefits of 10% weight loss

Mortality	>20% fall in total mortality
	>30% fall in diabetes-related deaths
	>40% fall in obesity-related deaths
Blood pressure	10 mmHg fall in systolic and diastolic pressure
Diabetes	50% fall in fasting glucose
Lipids	10% decrease in total cholesterol
	15% decrease in low-density lipoproteins (LDL)
	30% decrease in tryglycerides
	5% increase in high-density lipoproteins (HDL)

Source: Goldstein (1992)

but to date I am aware of no more than a dozen specialist centres. One example of such a specialist obesity clinic is at the University Hospital in Nottingham, where I work. In contrast, there are 36,000 general practitioners and 20,000 practice nurses. This is surely a resource that we can use to make a significant dent in this epidemic of obesity.

Obstacles to the management of obesity

Obesity is a medical problem and we have to accept that it is our problem, but there are several, very understandable, negative reasons why we may be reluctant to do so. We do not have the time, but neither do we have the knowledge or the training. Medical students generally receive minimal teaching on nutritional matters.

Obesity is a chronic disease. You cannot send the patient away with a single prescription and hope they are cured. They keep coming back, and if you are going to do anything about it, you have to acknowledge this fact and be prepared to see them, not just for 1 month, or 12 months, but year after year. Patients are frustrated by their return to pre-treatment weights, so are the doctors, so are the nurses. It is hard to accept that the fault may lie with us, and we tend to blame, not ourselves, but the patient.

Even if we measure our patients' weight routinely, as most of us are obliged to do when they first join our practice, it does not influence the way we manage obesity. We measure their height and their weight, the computer calculates the BMI and then we file it away and do no more about it. Just acknowledging that the BMI is raised is not enough – we must log it as a disease in its own right. The next practitioner who picks up that patient will then see this and be far more likely to address it as a medical issue.

The other problem is that we feel we have to produce patients like Alison, every time, because that is what patients expect. They want to look sylph-like, but, realistically, it does not always happen – often we struggle to help them lose even 10 per cent of their body weight. The good news, however, is that 10 per cent – even 5 per cent – is medically beneficial. We need to forget so-called 'ideal' weights and set patients a more realistic goal of 10 per cent weight loss over 3–6 months. If this more modest goal is reached, they will be happy and their doctors will feel that they have achieved something.

We need clear practical guidelines, such as those produced by the National Obesity Forum. General practitioners and primary care workers are unlikely to read a 13-page document on obesity management. We therefore condensed it to just one page. It simply tells general practitioners who they should be treating, and how. If anyone wants to look them up in full they are easily accessible on our web site at www.nationalobesityforum.org.uk.

It is quite clear that doctors and nurses and health visitors need, and indeed are asking for, readily accessible training in their own regions, but to date it is not being delivered. There is good evidence from the US, for example, that good quality education can actually make a difference. In Pittsburgh in 1997, some primary care physicians went on a 2-day intensive course on obesity – why it was a problem and what they should do about it. When they went back into practice, not only did the number of interventions double from 45 per cent to 89 per cent, but the quality of the interventions was much greater (Simkin-Silverman and Wing, 1997). The National Obesity Forum was initially set up to bring together those of us in primary care who wanted to do something about obesity, who have a keen interest in it, but did not necessarily know how to go about it. As a group, we hope to exert more influence over what happens in primary care, through government, health authorities and primary care trusts. We have also launched a national best practice initiative for obesity management, and we have extended our network to include all interested healthcare workers.

Managing obesity in primary care

How should obesity be managed in primary care? Realistically, with the time and resource constraints we have, we suggest focusing on those patients with a BMI greater than 30. Those with a BMI between 25 and 30 may be helped by commercial agencies or self-help groups, although most doctors could consider treatment if the patient presents as a self-referral. Many patients, however, do not ask for help. They may present with unrelated problems, and it is at this point that the problem of obesity can be identified and addressed. One of the advantages of primary care is that the patient and the patient's family are seen over many years, even decades, thus building up sufficient trust to allow us to raise the sensitive subject of obesity without offence.

To maximize this opportunity to help there has to be regular input, certainly on a monthly level – anything less than this will see the patient's enthusiasm dissipate very rapidly. I also ask them to commit themselves to at least 12 months of working together. One possibility might be a nurse-led clinic. A major problem with our present system is that the average general practitioner has only 8 minutes with each patient. This is one of the reasons we tend to send a lot of these patients to the practice nurse, because their appointment times may be more flexible.

In terms of management, use the guidelines, be they local or national, and use a combination of dietary restriction, physical activity, and behavioural change, but also, if necessary, medication. Patients with a BMI greater than 40 are the most resistant to treatment. You need to consider whether you can manage these yourself or whether you need to refer them to a specialist centre, should one be available. Surgery is even a possibility, and if you have that facility locally, consider referring these patients, particularly those who do not respond to normal conservative treatment.

Make sure patients are ready to make drastic changes to their lifestyle. If they are not ready to do so, it will not happen. Do not invest any time or effort in them, but explain why and invite them to come back when they are ready. Motivation is the key. Any weight loss achieved is likely to be in proportion to the enthusiasm and determination, both of the patient and of those who are helping them to lose weight.

Keep the advice simple. Telling a patient to reduce his or her calorific intake by 500 kcal is meaningless unless you are a dietitian. It is much easier to be told to reduce one's food intake by 20 per cent, which, for most of us, would lead to a 500-kcal deficit. Whatever we do, it has to be realistic, sustainable and not be too radical. Make any changes gradual – remember you are seeing them in a month and that this programme takes a year. You do not have to do it all in one day.

Physical activity is an absolutely crucial and indispensable part of any weight loss programme. Patients who exercise are not only more likely to lose weight, but to maintain that weight loss.

Exercise on prescription does not work. Newcastle tried this scheme with 523 patients over a 12-month period and it failed (Harland *et al.*, 1999). It is a well-known fact that a large number of people join a gym, at no mean expense, go three times and stop. It has been shown that home-based schemes are the most effective. Walking is perhaps dull but it is something patients can do on a daily basis, whether it is picking up the children from school or walking to work. They can walk at the weekend or on holiday and they can even start riding a bike – all simple measures, but cumulative. As far as diet is concerned, simple behavioural changes can help, such as eating in one room and making it the sole activity. Eating around the house, in front of the TV or while driving the car should be avoided as they only serve to increase our total consumption. Snacking in these circumstances must be replaced by other distractions, tailor-made to suit individual needs. Drugs are expensive and again they must be chosen to suit the individual patient. They can, however, help patients lose weight, and the benefits, I believe, are likely to outweigh the costs.

Why do patients want to lose weight? They do not generally ask for help in order to improve their diabetes, nor to improve their heart disease. They come, predominantly, for the following reasons. 'I want my kids to feel proud of me. I want to walk to school and not have other kids laugh at my kids because their mum is fat. I want to go swimming. I want to get a job. I want to travel on an aeroplane.' A 23-year-old lad once said to me, 'There are

350 students in my hall at university, that is, 349 normal ones and then me. That is why I want to lose weight.'

Childhood obesity is clearly an ever-increasing problem too. Both in North America and the UK, they are now finding children with type 2 diabetes, a disease hitherto only associated with overweight adults. Now it is appearing in overweight children. While we may criticize the way we manage adult diabetes by treating the symptoms and not the cause, in some ways we are guilty of the same thing with obesity. If we are seeing obese adults, it is because we have failed to address the problem in their childhood.

I would urge general practitioners to start to tackle obesity now in their own practices. You *can* help your patients achieve significant improvements in their physical wellbeing, in their psychological well being and in their future health. You can measure these benefits through weight loss, but they can also be measured through the psychological changes that follow. It is extremely gratifying.

References

Adami, H.O., Day, N.E., Tricopoulos, D. and Willett, W.C. (2001) Primary and secondary prevention in the reduction of cancer morbidity and mortality. *Eur J Cancer*, 37(Suppl. 8): S118–27.

Chan, J.M., Rimm, E.B., Colditz, G.A., Stampfer, M.J., Willett, W.C. *et al.* (1994) Obesity, fat distribution and weight gain as risk factors for clinical diabetes in men. *Diabetes Care*, 17: 961–9.

Goldstein, D. (1992) Beneficial health effects of modest weight loss. *Int J Obes*, 16: 397–415.

Harland, J., White, M., Drinkwater, C., Chinn, D., Farr, L. and Howel, D. (1999) The Newcastle exercise project: a randomised controlled trial of methods to promote physical activity in primary care. *Br Med J*, 319: 828–32.

National Audit Office (2001) *Tackling Obesity in England*. Report by the Controller and auditor general. London: The Stationery Office.

Pi-Sunyer, F. (1993) Medical hazards of obesity. *Ann Intern Med*, 119: 655–60.

Simkin-Silverman, L.R. and Wing, R.R. (1997) Management of obesity in primary care. *Obes. Res*, 5: 603–12.

Part IV
The challenge

8 Adult obesity: a paediatric challenge

David Hall

My interest is in preventative child health programmes and, in particular, in how the whole programme of disparate activities and aims hangs together. One topic that has had a lot of attention is growth monitoring, where the question arose as to whether we could, or should, be screening for growth disorders. Both the Child Growth Foundation and the paediatric endocrinologists were very anxious to do so, yet most such disorders affect children relatively rarely, in the region of one or two per 5,000 children. There is also evidence that most short children are not unduly distressed by their size, whereas many overweight children are. Perhaps it is time to switch the focus of our attention.

There have been lengthy discussions in relation to stature as to whether a single measurement would identify children with a growth disorder, or whether one would need serial measurements, over a period of time. It was clear that if measurements were to be made, they had to be both accurate and reliable, otherwise it would be impossible to distinguish growth from the background or statistical noise. It is also important to understand what is to be done with the information obtained. All too often in the history of community child health, data have been collected without any clear idea as to what is to be done with the results. Exactly the same rules apply if the intention is to identify the child who is beginning to develop a weight problem.

Last July, the Child Growth Foundation sponsored a workshop on obesity and it was clear that most paediatricians had a lot to learn about the causes and health consequences of obesity. There was also debate as to whether obesity might be considered as a target for a screening programme and, finally, discussion as to what other initiatives might be appropriate and feasible within the sphere of public health. The conclusion was that obesity is a major problem and requires a multi-dimensional and multi-disciplinary approach.

Faced with a serious but common problem, such as obesity, there are three possible approaches. The first is the standard medical approach – the consultation or problem solving model, such as a general practitioner might adopt. The second approach is to screen and thus identify the problem at an early stage before it develops further. The third approach is prevention – to stop it happening at all through a public health or health promotion strategy. All three of these strands have an important role to play, but prevention is clearly the ultimate goal.

As far as screening is concerned, it might be possible to involve general practitioners or school nurses. Serial measurements of height and weight, a form of screening, would check for a rising body mass index (BMI), and an additional measure, such as a waist measurement, could even be added in order to identify children most at risk. The rationale for screening is early detection and the prevention of extreme degrees of overweight.

Screening carries a particular responsibility and many have argued that when you take the action to the client, rather than the other way round, the ethical imperatives are very different. The obligation to get it right is that much greater. When the customer or patient asks for help, one does the best one can, but when unsolicited advice is offered to an apparently healthy person, the imperative to be correct is that much greater. A classic example was the advice given, without good evidence, as to the best sleeping position for the prevention of cot death. It took 25 years to realize that totally the wrong advice had been given, because it was never based on any sound research, and it undoubtedly cost the lives of many babies. It is a lesson worth remembering, before rushing to implement any new public health initiative designed to make everybody healthier – it must be evidence-based.

Screening may well appear cheap, but it is, in fact, very expensive. When calculations are made as to how many lives are actually saved per pound spent, the equation can look very different. The rules with regard to screening have to be, and indeed are, very strict. Muir Gray, a leading proponent of rational screening policy maintains that the balance of good and harm in most screening programmes is a very fine one. He has also been heard to remark that we should not be interested in whether screening works in the hands of a keen researcher, but whether it will work on a wet Thursday afternoon in Ambridge.

In brief, our conference concluded that currently BMI measurement does not fulfil all the criteria required to be used in a screening programme, as laid down by the Children's Group of the National Screening Committee. The most compelling reason concerns treatment. One of the criteria for screening is that there should be some intervention, of proven effectiveness, acceptable to the population and importantly, facilities to provide the treatment to all those identified. The unanimous view among paediatricians is that it is extraordinarily difficult to achieve significant weight reduction, even in the highly motivated, self-referred child with strong family support.

Very often, one does well just to control further weight gain. To expect children revealed by a school screening process to participate in all the rigours of a weight reduction programme, when it works with such difficulty for the highly motivated self-referred child, seems optimistic in the extreme.

The second criterion is that all other ways of approaching the problem should first be considered before deciding to invest resources in a screening programme. In the case of obesity, this avenue may not have been fully explored. There is still much research to be done, for example, in relation to appetite and its control.

Obesity is a major problem for the children concerned, and a challenge for general practitioners, paediatricians, and all health professionals. It needs to be tackled with all the tools at our disposal, but for the present, looking at it from a public health angle, the approach is not that of screen and treat. Of course, so long as routine height and weight measurements continue to be made at school entry, for example, in order to identify obvious growth disorders, individual children with a whole range of growth problems, including severe obesity, will be identified on clinical grounds – but obesity is not the main target of these measurements at the present time.

As far as the BMI of school entrants is concerned, we see its main value as a measure of public health, both a record of the status quo and a tool with which to monitor changes in the health of the nation. This approach does, however, require several caveats. One of the first rules, as implied earlier, is do no harm. It is conceivable that the increase in anorexia and other eating disorders, now so widespread, has been triggered by the high profile given to obesity. It is just as likely, however, that the problems with such disorders are simply rising in parallel with, and independently of, the rise in obesity and need not be attributed to any health professional initiatives.

The second public health issue to be considered is the single versus the multi-pronged approach. Tackling obesity in isolation is not necessarily the most efficient approach. We all have our particular areas of interest, and the evidence seems to be that many of the measures that might be adopted to prevent or reduce obesity would also benefit many other areas of health, from osteoporosis to cardiovascular disease. This multi-focused approach seems to be the most effective, and is particularly valuable in the field of school health promotion, where to focus on a single undesirable characteristic can be stigmatizing, to say the least, for the child concerned.

The third question is how to actually implement an agreed approach. How does one convince individuals, and organizations in particular, of the need to change? To date, we have signally failed to induce any sense of urgency in any official pronouncements.

Ideally, we should be trying to create a sense of urgency amongst the population as a whole. We should be giving them the message that most of us would benefit from a 10 per cent or even 5 per cent weight loss. The classic argument, it has been said, is that one should not really ask if a person has a disease, but how much of it they have got. Increasingly, the public health strategy in this and other areas of child development is not to target particular individuals, but rather to shift the population mean, so that everyone benefits. Instead of focusing on the slow talking child, there has been a call for measures to be put in place that will help *all* parents improve their children's language acquisition. This could be the most relevant philosophy in tackling rising levels of obesity.

Community-wide approaches that could be considered in the public health arena include improvements in ante-natal care, breastfeeding figures, infant and toddler diets and television viewing habits. Changing behaviour is difficult though not impossible. Successes in public health include drink driving and seat belts (though this required legislation), sudden infant death syndrome (simple advice to turn the baby), poisoning (new packaging), and immunization (benefits greater than risks). Relative failures include smoking, breast-feeding, eating habits, cycling to work (figures could improve, given more cycle lanes).

Recent pronouncements from ministers at the Departments of Health and of Education and Skills do suggest that there is a growing awareness in Government that obesity is a serious problem. Policies are beginning to emerge that may address the intertwined problems of eating behaviour and physical activity. A conference hosted by the National Audit Office (http://www.nao.gov.uk/) in 2002 brought together a range of contributors and there seemed to be reason for optimism that obesity is at last moving up the agenda for improving the health of the nation.

Index